Dental Embryology, Histology, AND Anatomy

THIRD EDITION

MARY BATH-BALOGH, BA, BS, MS

Instructor, Anatomy and Physiology
Department of Biology
Pierce College Fort Steilacom
Lakewood, Washington

MARGARET J. FEHRENBACH, RDH, MS

Oral Biologist and Dental Hygienist
Adjunct Instructor, BASDH Degree Program
St. Petersburg College
St. Petersburg, Florida

Educational Consultant and Dental Technical Writer
Seattle, Washington

ELSEVIER
SAUNDERS

ELSEVIER
SAUNDERS

3251 Riverport Lane
St. Louis, Missouri 63043

**WORKBOOK ILLUSTRATED DENTAL EMBRYOLOGY,
HISTOLOGY, AND ANATOMY**

ISBN: 978-1-4377-2510-0

International Standard Book Number 978-1-4377-2510-0

Acquisitions Editor: Kristin Hebberd
Developmental Editor: Joslyn Dumas
Publishing Services Manager: Gayle May
Project Manager: Mahalakshmi Nithyanand

Printed in United States of America

Last digit is the print number: 9 8 7 6 5 4 3 2 1

PREFACE

This companion to *Illustrated Dental Embryology, Histology, and Anatomy* provides a wide range of activities and skill-building exercises to strengthen student readers' understanding of the principles discussed in the main textbook. The companion includes graph paper templates and evaluation criteria to help when drawing teeth. It also has structure identification exercises, glossary exercises, case studies, information on infection control and occlusal evaluation, and removable tooth identification flash cards. A special thanks to Pat Thomas, CMI for her contributions to the first edition art program. Her work has been truly beneficial to this text.

Additional material for students can be found online on the associated Evolve website, including answers to the Workbook's glossary exercises. We hope that this material will help students integrate their knowledge more easily into clinical dental coursework.

Mary Bath-Balogh
Margaret J. Fehrenbach

CONTENTS

Structure

Identification

Exercises

UNIT I: REVIEW OF DENTAL STRUCTURES

Chapter 1: Face and Neck Regions

Directions: Check off the items noted during an extraoral examination of a peer. Standard precautions and personal protection equipment (PPE) must be used. The patient should be seated in an upright position. Good lighting and exposure of the area being assessed are essential (e.g., collar and tie loosened, glasses removed); use both visual inspection and palpation. Include also the lymph nodes of the face and neck, if applicable.

Regions of the Face	
Frontal, Orbital, and Nasal Regions	
Forehead	
Orbits	
External Nose: Root of Nose, Apex of Nose, Nares, Nasal Septum, Nasal Alae	
Infraorbital Zygomatic Regions	
Zygomatic Arches	
Temporomandibular Joints	
Buccal Regions	
Masseter Muscles	
Angles of the Mandible	
Parotid Salivary Glands	
Oral Region	
Lips: Vermilion Zone and Border	
Philtrum	
Tubercle of Upper Lip	
Labial Commissures	

Structure Identification Exercise for Chapter 1: Face and Neck Regions (*continued*):

Mental Region and Lower Face	
Mandible: Rami, Coronoid Processes, Coronoid Notches, Mandibular Condyles, Mandibular Notches	
Regions of the Neck	
Sternocleidomastoid Muscles	
Hyoid Bone	
Thyroid Cartilage	
Thyroid Gland	
Submandibular Salivary Glands	
Sublingual Salivary Glands	

Chapter 2: Oral Cavity and Pharynx

Directions: Check off the items noted during an intraoral examination of a peer. Standard precautions and personal protection equipment (PPE) must be used. The patient should be seated in a dental chair in a supine position; use preprocedural antimicrobial mouth rinse, remove any pigmented lipsticks, and apply non-petroleum lubricant to cracked and dry areas; remove any removable appliances. Using visual inspection and palpation, make sure to also note normal variations such as Fordyce's spots, linea alba, exostoses, mandibular tori, and a palatal torus, if applicable. The base of the tongue and its structures, such as the lingual tonsil, are usually not visible when examining the oral cavity; however, note the relationship of the nasopharynx and laryngopharynx to the oropharynx. When examining mucosal surfaces, it is important to gently dry those surfaces with a gauze or air syringe, so that color or texture changes will become more obvious.

Oral Cavity	
Oral Vestibules	
Labial Mucosa	
Buccal Mucosa and Buccal Fat Pads	
Parotid Papillae	
Parotid Salivary Glands	
Vestibular Fornix	
Alveolar Mucosa and Mucobuccal Folds	
Labial Frenum: Maxillary and Mandibular	

Structure Identification Exercise for Chapter 2: Oral Cavity and Pharynx (*continued*):

Jaws, Alveolar Processes, Teeth, and Dental Arches	
Maxilla: Maxillary Sinuses, Alveolar Processes, Canine Eminences, Maxillary Teeth, Maxillary Tuberosities	
Mandible: Alveolar Processes, Canine Eminences, Mandibular Teeth, Retromolar Pads	
Teeth: Crown, Enamel, Anterior Teeth, Posterior Teeth, Incisors, Canines, Premolars, and Molars	
Gingiva and Associated Structures	
Attached Gingiva	
Mucogingival Junction	
Marginal Gingiva	
Gingival Sulci (location only)	
Interdental Gingiva	
Oral Cavity Proper	
Fauces	
Anterior Faucial Pillars	
Posterior Faucial Pillars	
Palatine Tonsils (if present)	
Palate	
Hard Palate	
Median Palatine Raphe	
Incisive Papilla	
Palatine Rugae	
Uvula of the Palate	
Soft Palate	
Pterygomandibular Folds	
Tongue	
Base of Tongue (anterior portion only)	
Body of Tongue	
Dorsal Surface	
Median Lingual Sulcus	
Filiform Lingual Papillae	
Sulcus Terminalis and Foramen Cecum (if possible)	

Structure Identification Exercise for Chapter 2: Oral Cavity and Pharynx (*continued*):

Circumvallate Lingual Papillae	
Lateral Surfaces	
Foliate Lingual Papillae	
Ventral Surface	
Plicae Fimbriatae	
Floor of the Mouth	
Lingual Frenum	
Sublingual Folds	
Sublingual Salivary Glands	
Submandibular Salivary Glands	
Sublingual Caruncles	
Pharynx	
Oropharynx	

UNIT II: DENTAL EMBRYOLOGY

Chapter 3: Overview of Prenatal Development

1. Figure 3-4

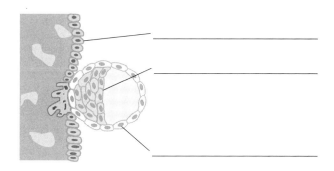

2. Figure 3-6

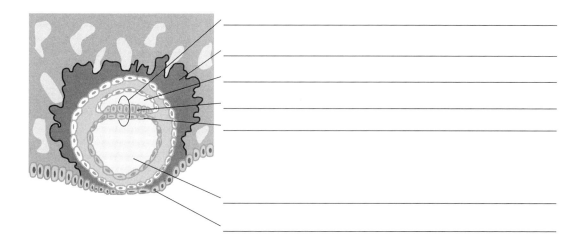

3. Figure 3-7

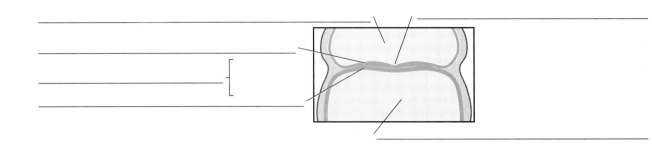

4. Figure 3-8

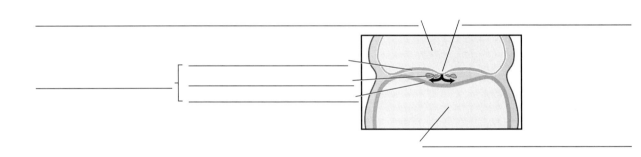

5. Figure 3-9

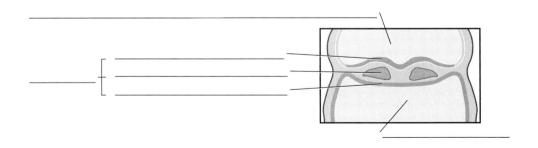

6.   Figure 3-10, *A*

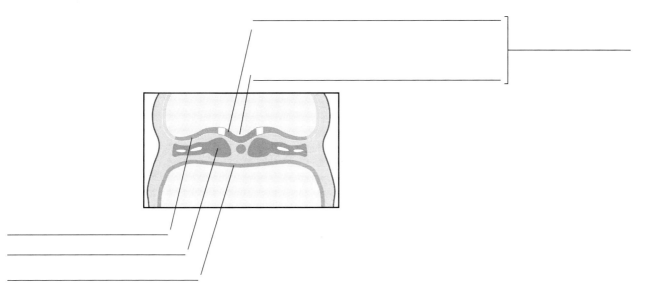

7.   Figure 3-10, *B*

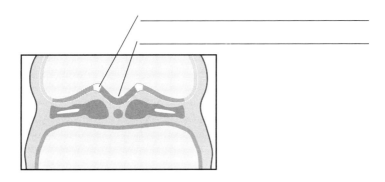

8.   Figure 3-10, *C*

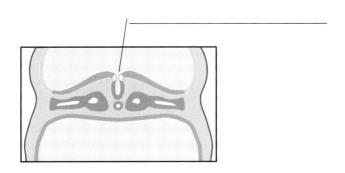

9. Figure 3-11, *A*

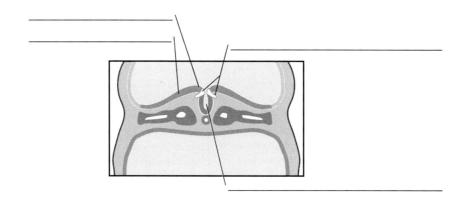

10. Figure 3-11, *B*

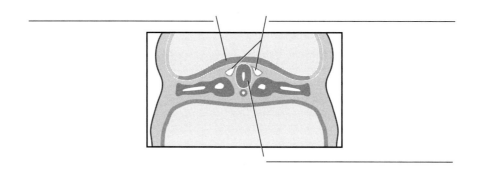

11. Figure 3-15

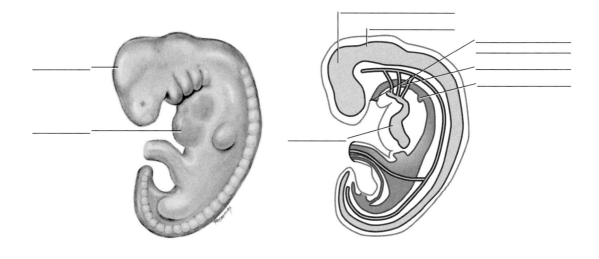

Chapter 4: Development of the Face and Neck

12. Figure 4-1

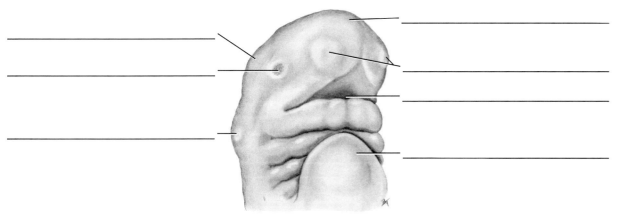

13. Figure 4-3

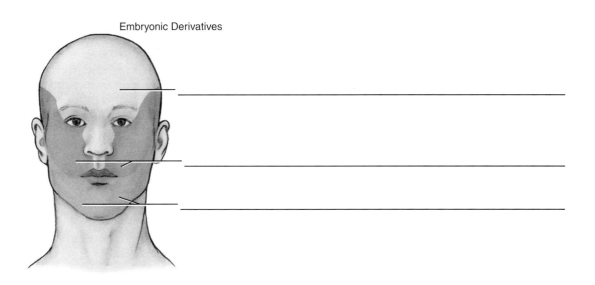

Embryonic Derivatives

14. Figure 4-5

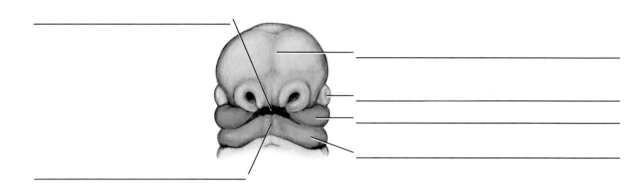

15. Figure 4-6

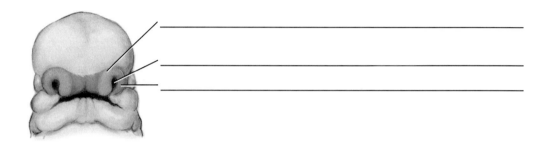

Chapter 5: Development of Orofacial Structures

16.   Figure 5-2

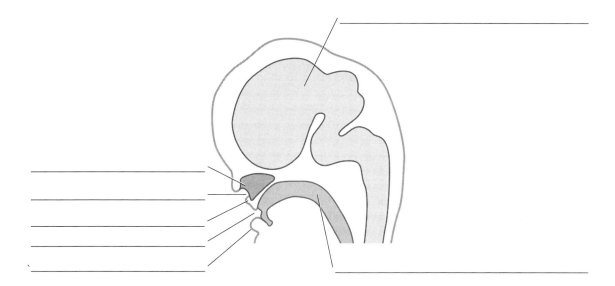

17.   Figure 5-3

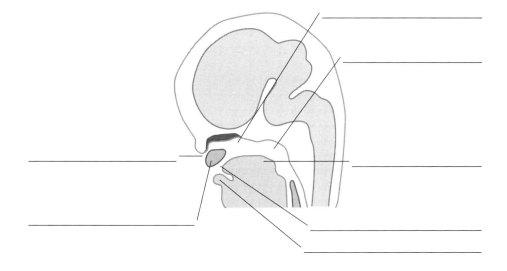

18. Figure 5-4, *A*

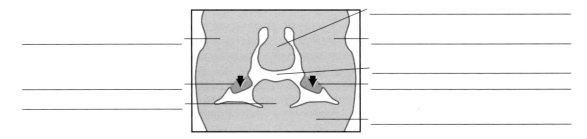

19. Figure 5-4, *C*

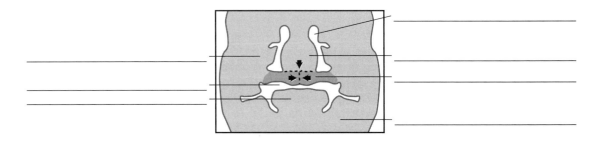

20. Figure 5-6

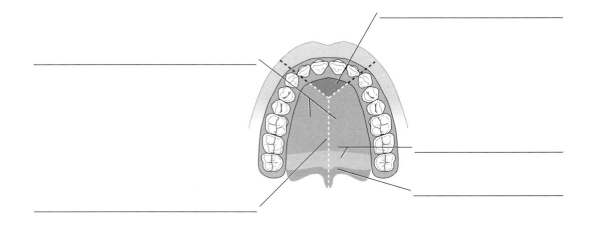

21. Figure 5-10, *A*

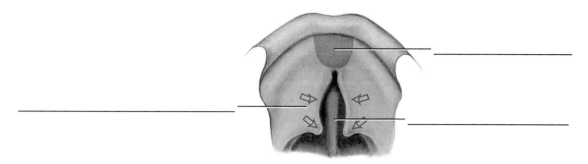

22. Figure 5-10, *B*

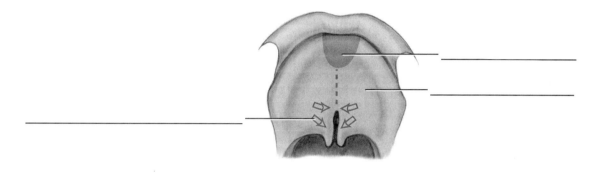

23. Figure 5-10, *C*

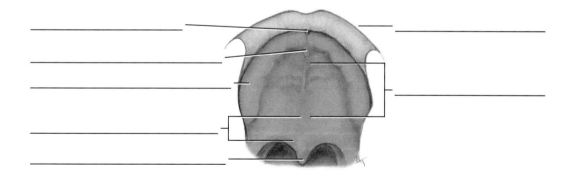

Chapter 6: Tooth Development and Eruption

24. Figure 6-2

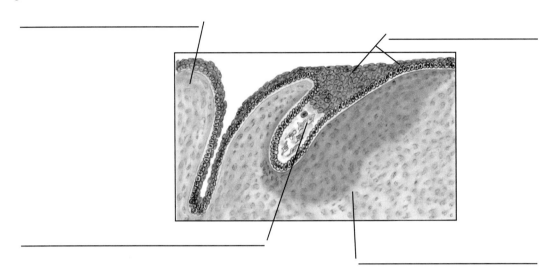

25. Figure 6-3

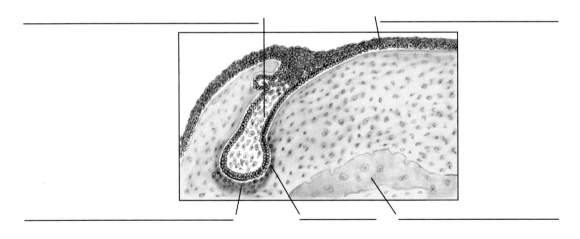

26. Figure 6-5

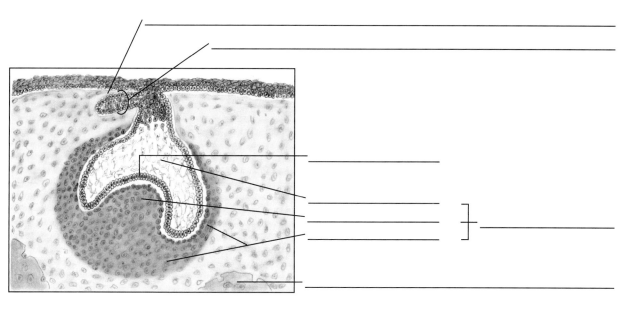

27. Figure 6-7

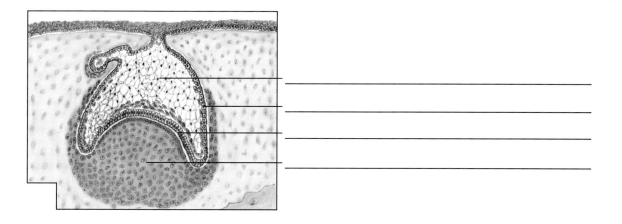

28. Figure 6-7

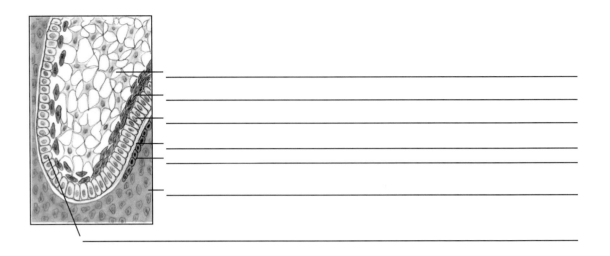

29. Figure 6-12

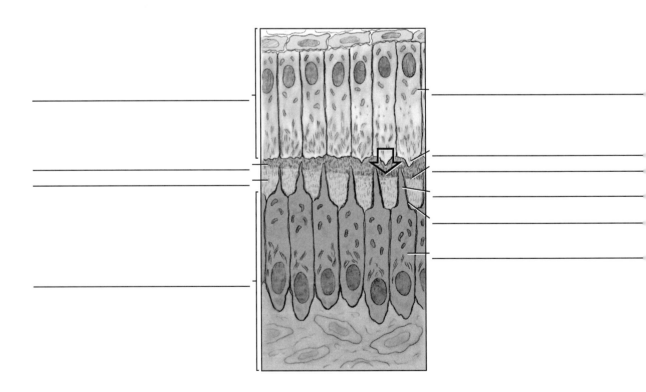

30. Figure 6-13

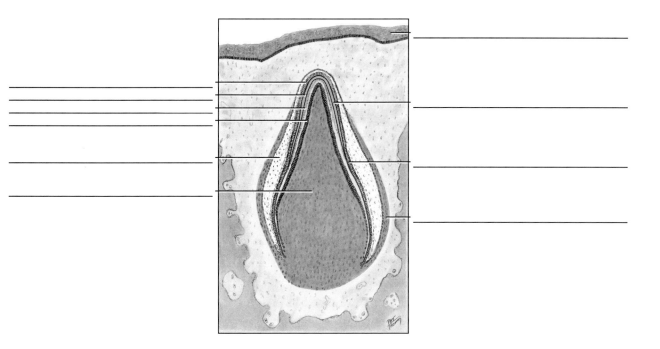

31. Figure 6-18, *A*

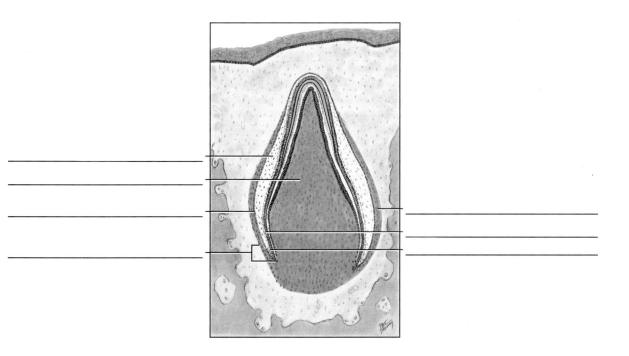

32. Figure 6-18, *B*

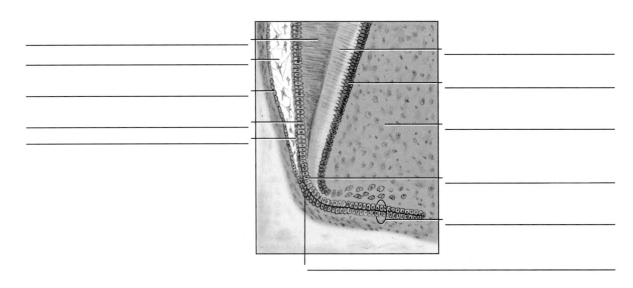

33. Figure 6-19

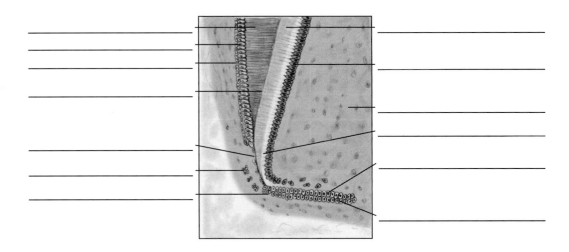

34. Figure 6-20

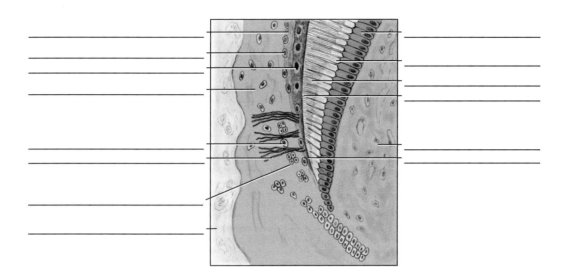

35. Figure 6-26

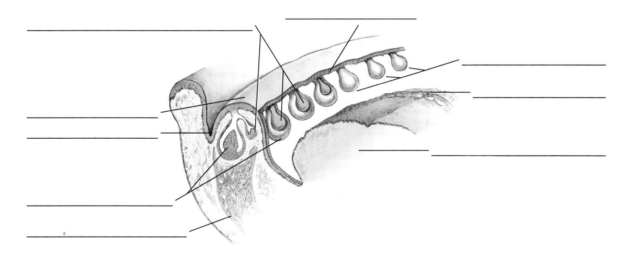

UNIT III: DENTAL HISTOLOGY

Chapter 7: Overview of the Cell

1. Figure 7-2

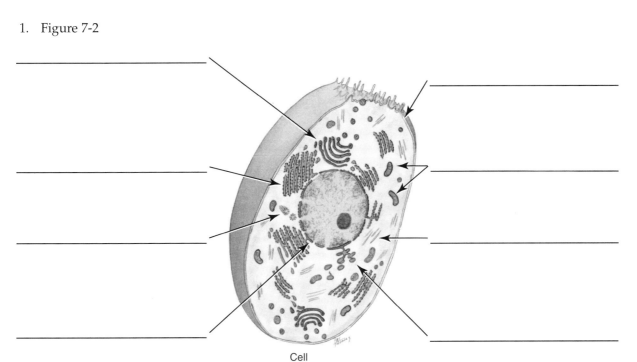

Cell

2. Figure 7-3

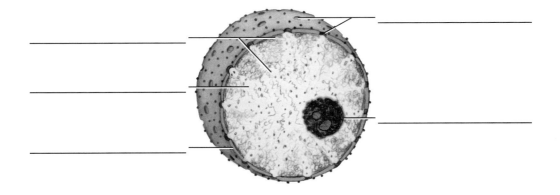

Chapter 8: Basic Tissues

3. Figure 8-4

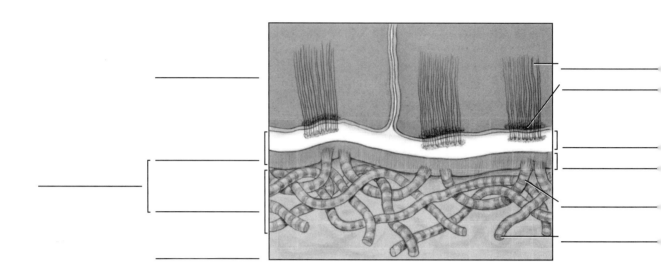

4. Figure 8-7

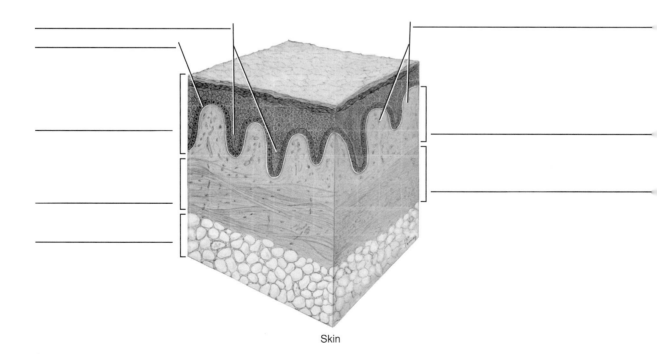

Skin

5. Figure 8-8

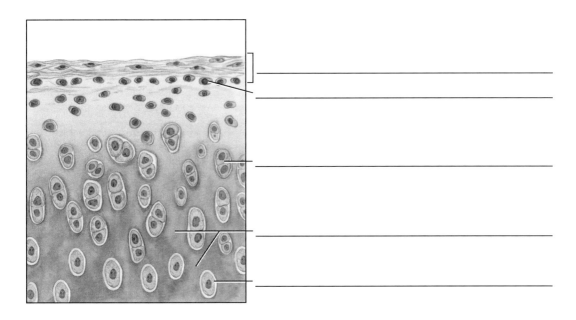

6. Figure 8-9

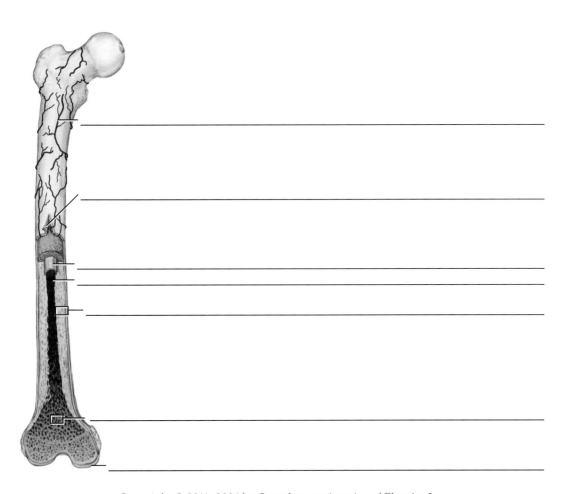

7. Figure 8-10

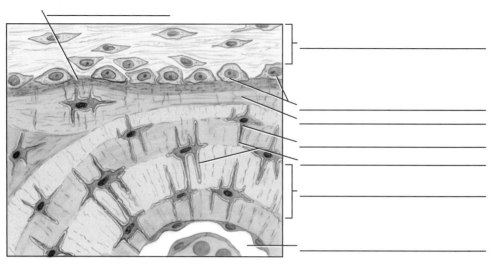

Diagram of the Histology of Bone

8. Figure 8-15

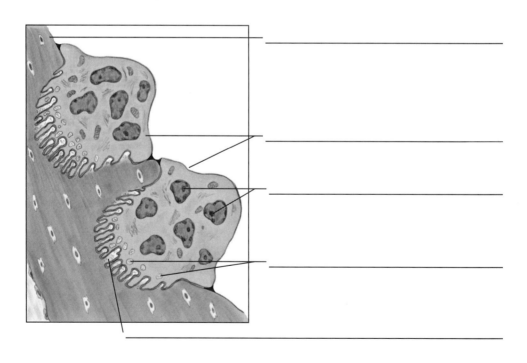

Chapter 9: Oral Mucosa

9.   Figure 9-1

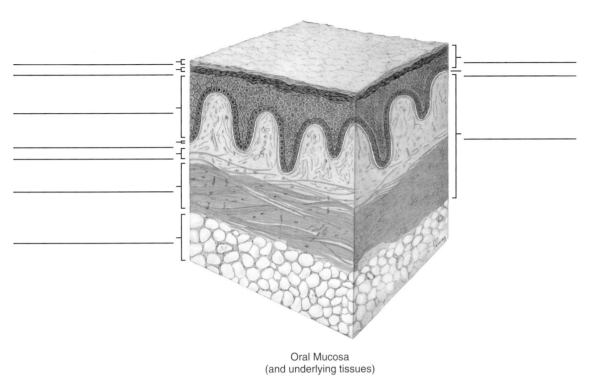

Oral Mucosa
(and underlying tissues)

10.   Figure 9-2

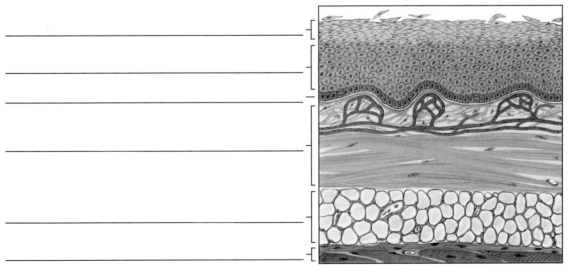

Nonkeratinized Stratified Squamous Epithelium
(and deeper tissues)

11. Figure 9-3

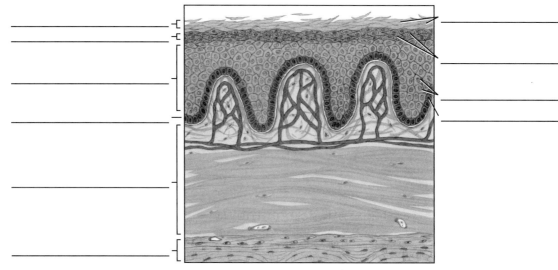

Orthokeratinized Stratified Squamous Epithelium
(and deeper tissues)

12. Figure 9-5

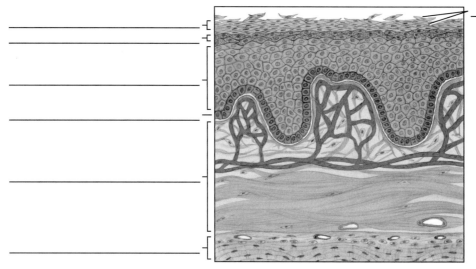

Parakeratinized Stratified Squamous Epithelium
(and deeper tissues)

13. Figure 9-7

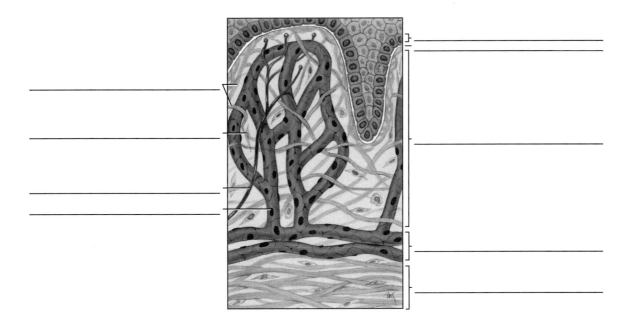

14. Figure 9-12

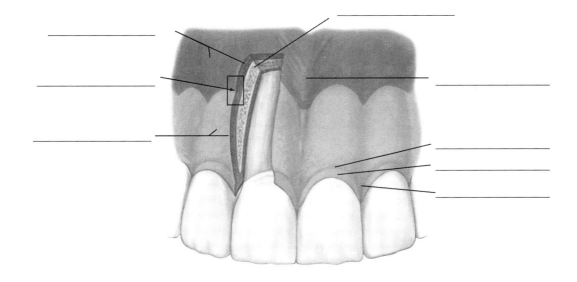

14.   Figure 9-12 (continued)

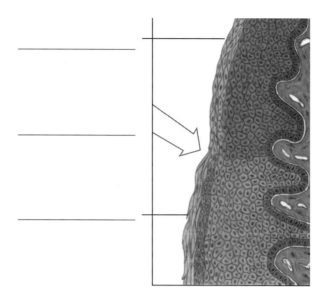

15.   Figure 9-16

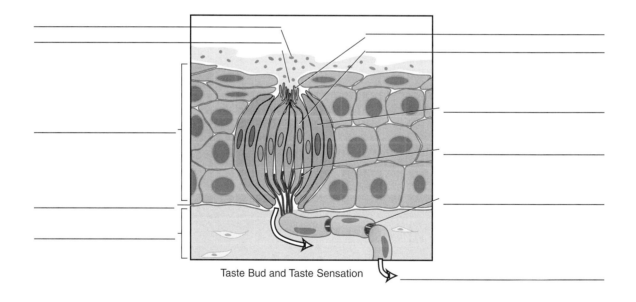

Taste Bud and Taste Sensation

Chapter 10: Gingival and Dentogingival Junctional Tissues

16. Figure 10-1

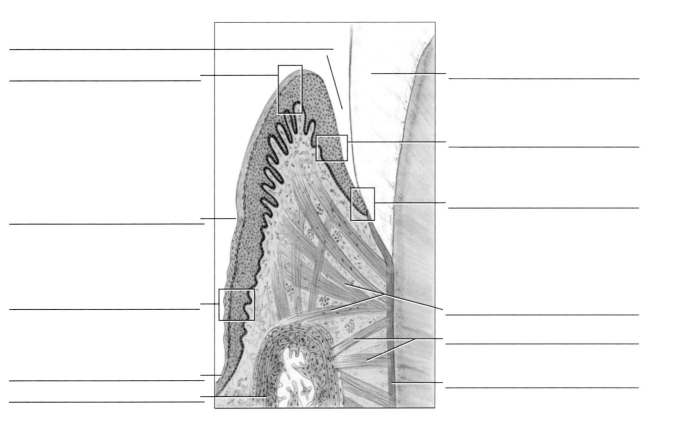

17. Figure 10-8

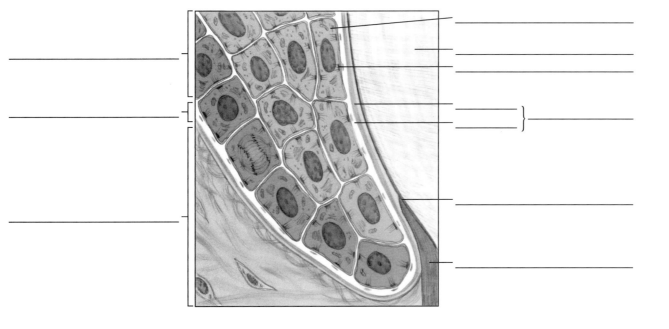

Chapter 11: Head and Neck Structures

18.   Figure 11-1, *B*

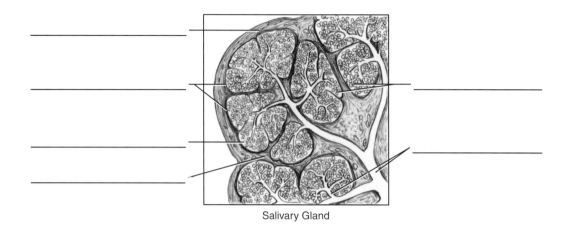

Salivary Gland

19.   Figure 11-6

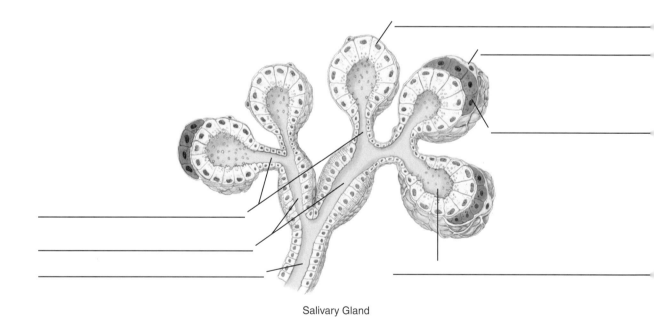

Salivary Gland

20. Figure 11-12, *B*

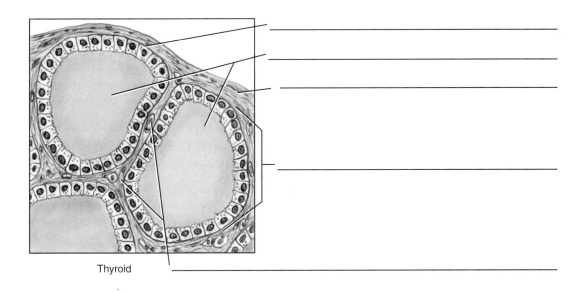

Thyroid

21. Figure 11-15, *A*

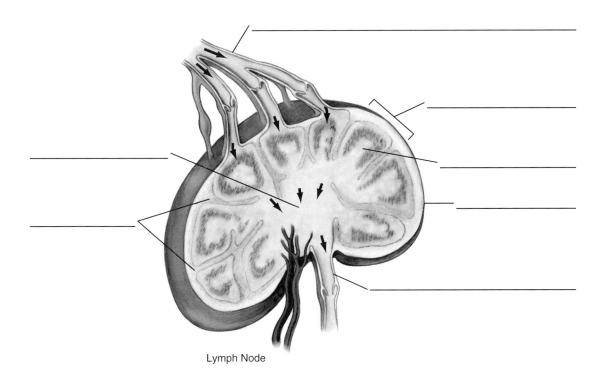

Lymph Node

22.   Figure 11-16, *A*

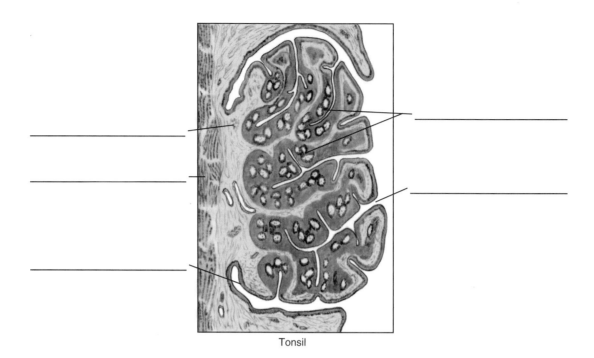

Tonsil

23.   Figure 11-19

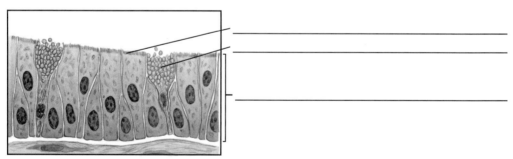

Nasal Cavity

Chapter 12: Enamel

24. Figure 12-6, *A*

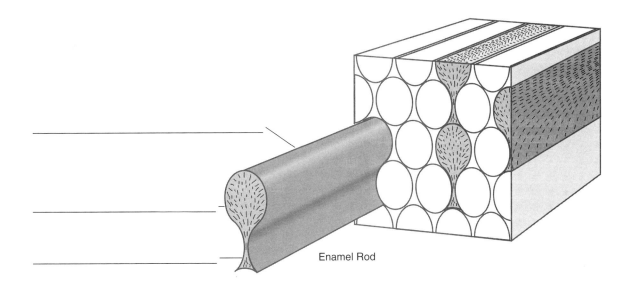

Enamel Rod

Chapter 13: Dentin and Pulp

25. Figure 13-11, Figure 13-16

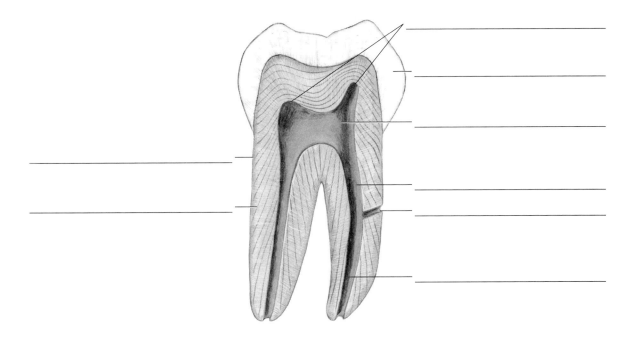

Chapter 14: Periodontium

26. Figure 14-1

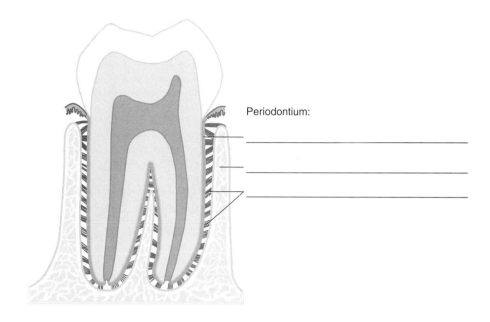

Periodontium:

_____

_____

_____

27. Figure 14-2

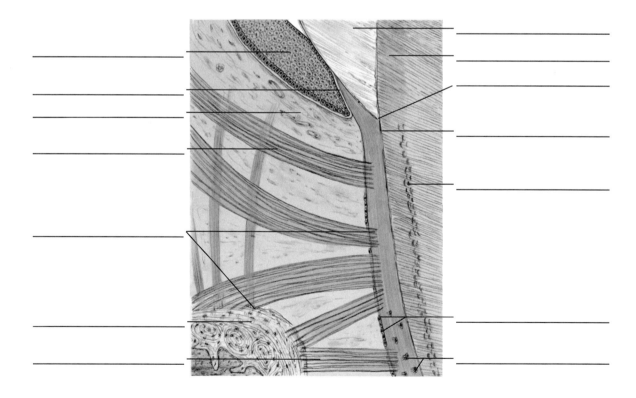

28. Figure 14-14

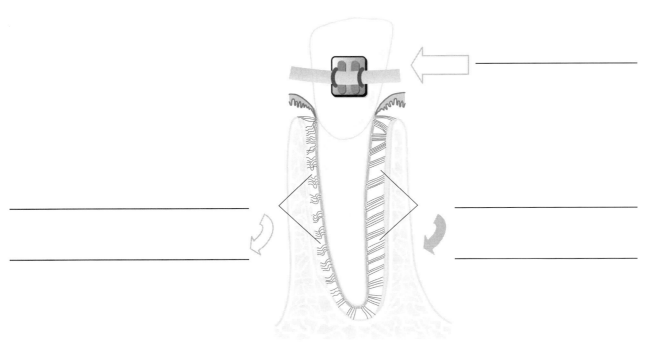

Orthodontic Tooth Movement

29. Figure 14-27

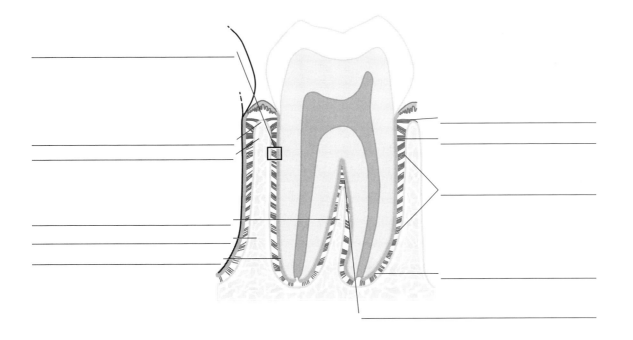

30. Figure 14-31

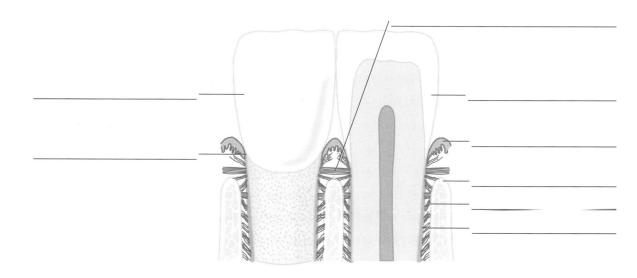

31. Figure 14-32

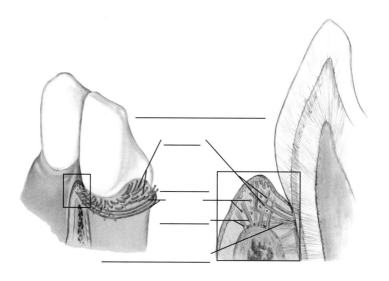

UNIT IV: DENTAL ANATOMY

Chapter 15: Overview of Dentitions

1. Figure 15-1

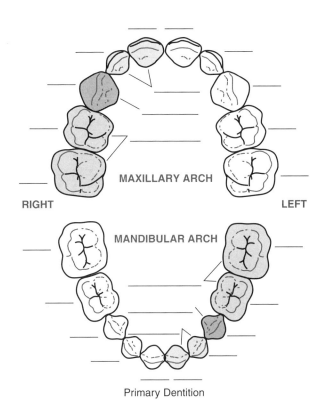

RIGHT   MAXILLARY ARCH   LEFT

MANDIBULAR ARCH

Primary Dentition

2. Figure 15-2

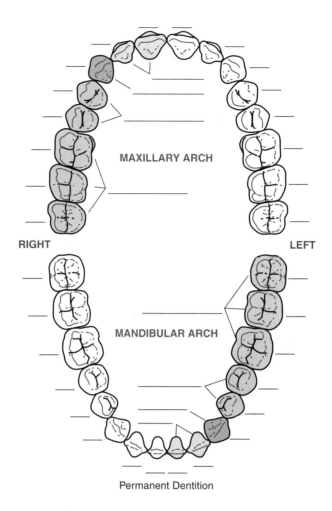

Permanent Dentition

3. Figure 15-5

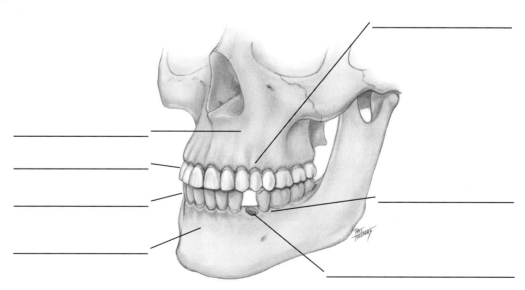

4. Figure 15-6

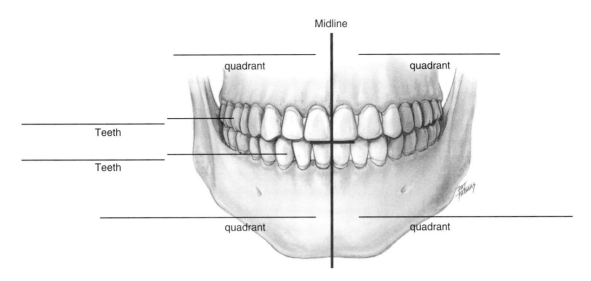

5. Figure 15-7

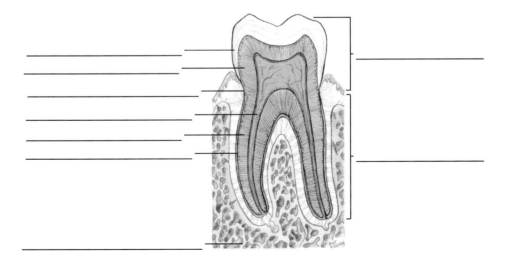

6. Figure 15-8

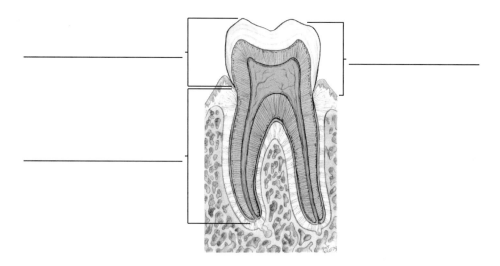

7. Figure 15-9

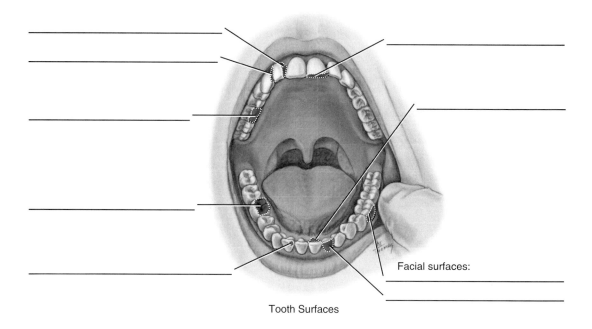

Facial surfaces:

Tooth Surfaces

8. Figure 15-12 (first)

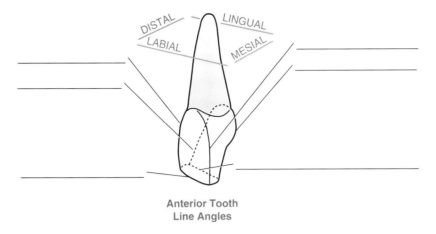

**Anterior Tooth
Line Angles**

9. Figure 15-12 (second)

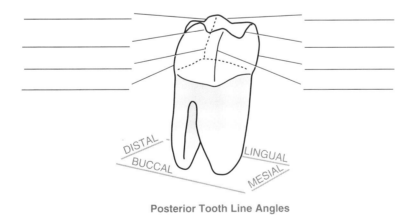

Posterior Tooth Line Angles

10. Figure 15-14 (first)

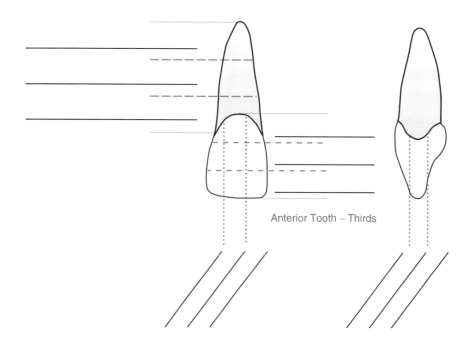

Anterior Tooth – Thirds

11. Figure 15-14 (second)

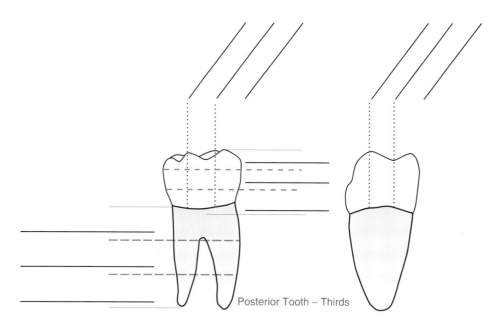

Posterior Tooth – Thirds

Chapter 16: Permanent Anterior Teeth

12. Figure 16-7 (first)

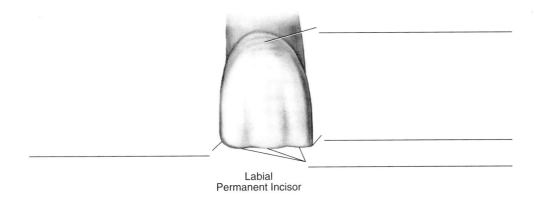

Labial
Permanent Incisor

13. Figure 16-7 (second)

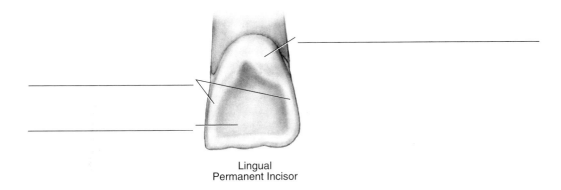

Lingual
Permanent Incisor

14. Figure 16-7 (third)

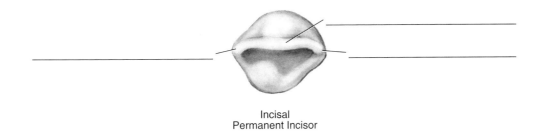

Incisal
Permanent Incisor

15. Figure 16-16

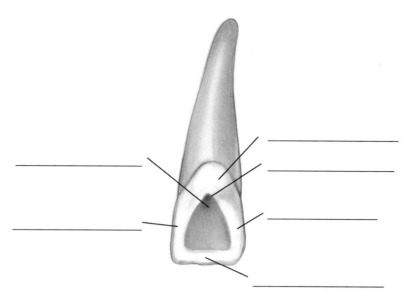

Permanent Maxillary Right Lateral Incisor

16. Figure 16-22

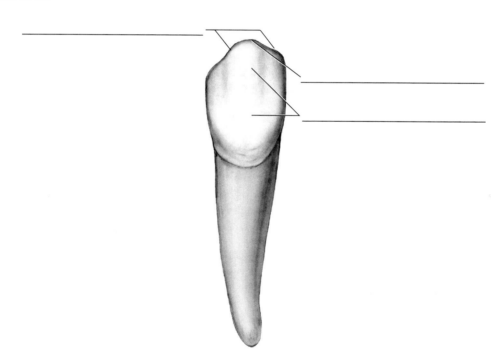

Labial View
Permanent Mandibular Right Canine

17. Figure 16-23

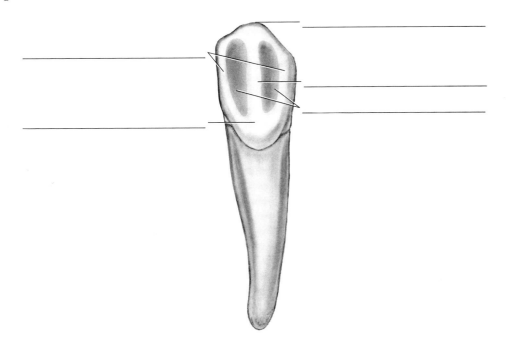

Lingual View
Permanent Mandibular Right Canine

18. Figure 16-27

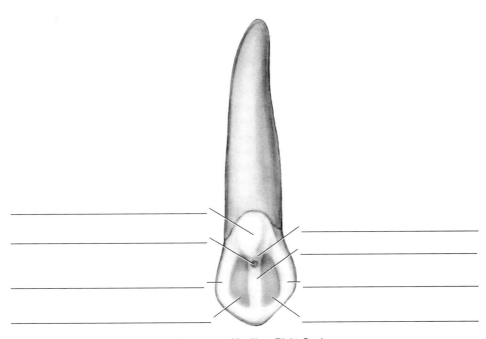

Permanent Maxillary Right Canine

Chapter 17: Permanent Posterior Teeth

19. Figure 17-2

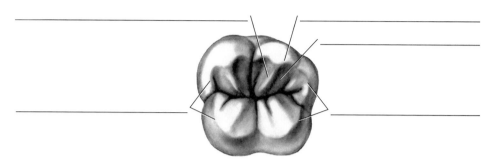

Permanent Posterior Tooth

20. Figure 17-4

Developmental grooves:

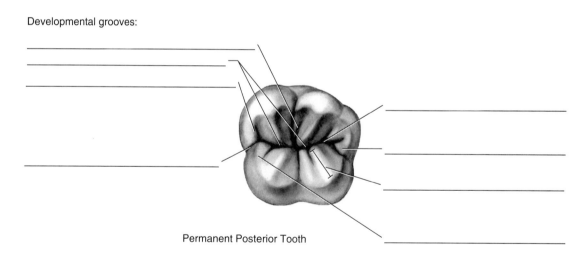

Permanent Posterior Tooth

21. Figure 17-13

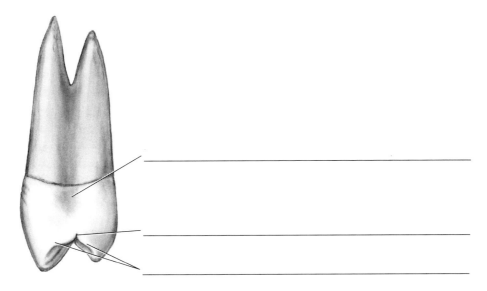

Permanent Maxillary Right First Premolar – Mesial View

22. Figure 17-14

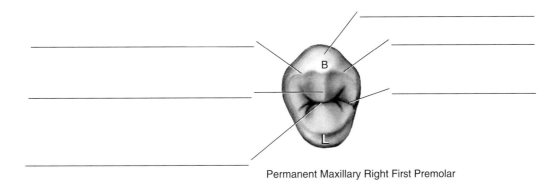

Permanent Maxillary Right First Premolar

23. Figure 17-15

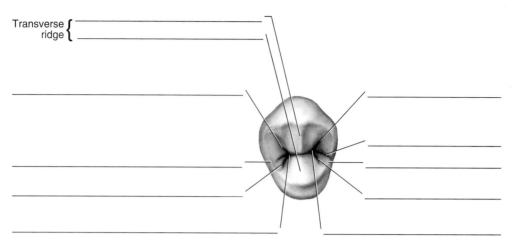

Transverse { ridge {

Permanent Maxillary Right First Premolar

24. Figure 17-33

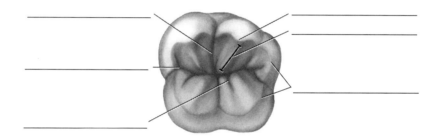

25. Figure 17-34 (first)

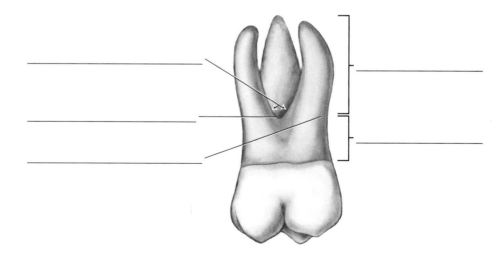

26. Figure 17-34 (second)

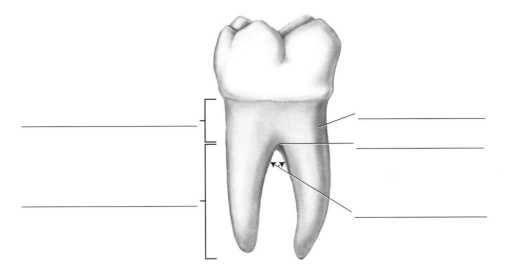

27. Figure 17-41

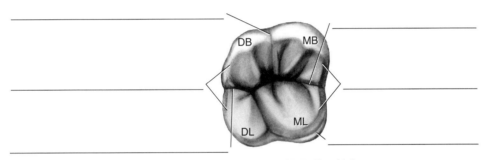

Permanent Maxillary Right First Molar

28. Figure 17-42

Central groove {

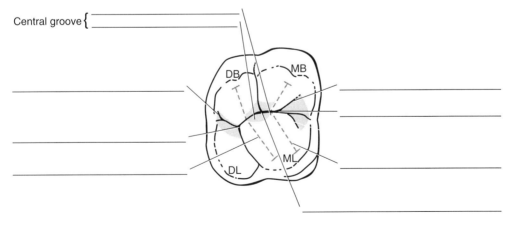

Permanent Maxillary Right First Molar

29. Figure 17-53

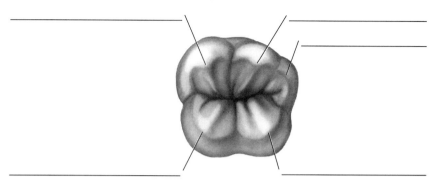

Permanent Mandibular Right First Molar

30. Figure 17-54

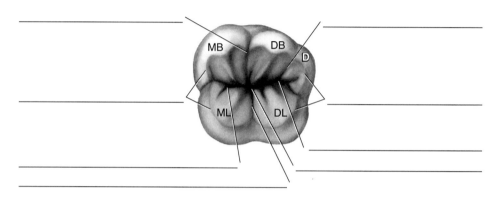

Permanent Mandibular Right First Molar

31. Figure 17-59

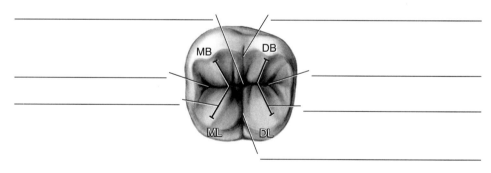

Permanent Mandibular Right Second Molar

Chapter 18: Primary Dentition

32.   Figure 18-3

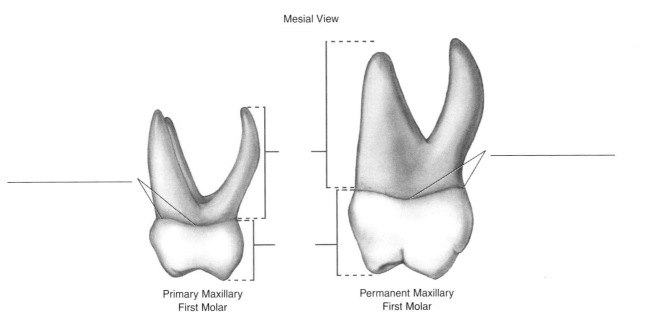

Mesial View

Primary Maxillary
First Molar

Permanent Maxillary
First Molar

Chapter 19: Temporomandibular Joint

33. Figure 19-1

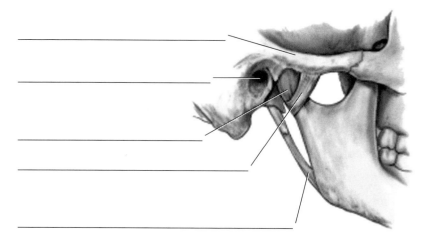

Temporomandibular Joint

34. Figure 19-5

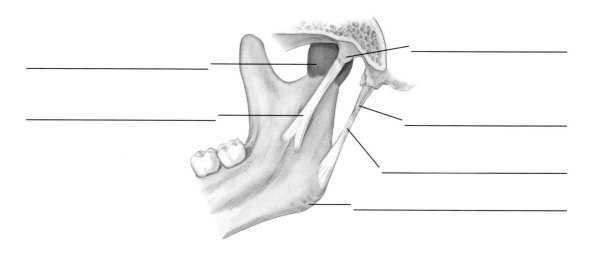

35. Figure 19-6

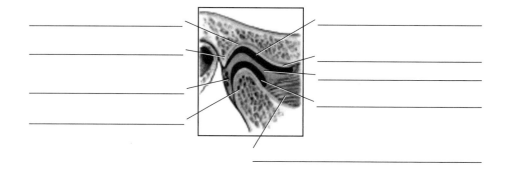

Chapter 20: Occlusion

36. Figure 20-2 (first)

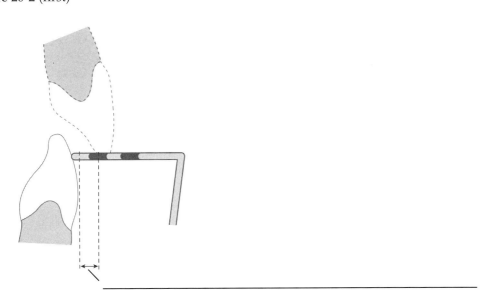

37. Figure 20-2 (second)

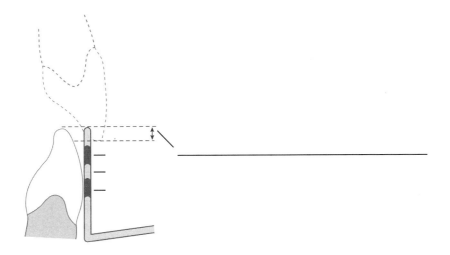

38. Figure 20-22

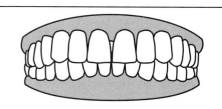

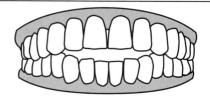

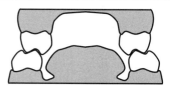

Posterior (bilateral)

 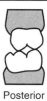

Anterior   Posterior

Glossary

Exercises

CHAPTER
WORD JUMBLES

CHAPTER 1

1. *Lower jaw* LEDIBMAN □□□□□□□
2. *Ramus part* ONORIDCO □□□□□□□
3. *Kisser corner* SUREMISCOM □□□□□□□□□
4. *Muscle mania* TERSEMAS □□□□□□□
5. *In thyroid* DOIRTHYARAP □□□□□□□□□□
6. *Cheeky gland* TIDROPA □□□□□□□
7. *Midline thickening* UERBCLET □□□□□□□□
8. *Lip place* TURIMLPH □□□□□□□□
9. *Head joint* MANBTOROPDIULAREM □□□□□□□□□□□□□□□□□
10. *Lip borders* LIONMIREV □□□□□□□□

CHAPTER 2

1. *Misplaced oil* ODRCYEF □□□□□□□
2. *Dog teeth* NESNICA □□□□□□□
3. *Grinding fun* CASTIMIOATN □□□□□□□□□□
4. *Arch bumps* SESXTOESO □□□□□□□□□
5. *Tooth padding* VAINGGI □□□□□□□
6. *Entrance walls* UFALAIC □□□□□□□
7. *Tongue specials* LALAPPIE □□□□□□□□

8. *Tongue line-up* VALARICTMUCLE ⬜⬜⬜⬜⬜⬜⬜⬜⬜⬜⬜⬜⬜

9. *Bony arches* EORVALAL ⬜⬜⬜⬜⬜⬜⬜⬜

10. *Mushroom shape* GORMFUNIF ⬜⬜⬜⬜⬜⬜⬜⬜⬜

CHAPTER 3

1. *Cavity fluid* TICNAIMO ⬜⬜⬜⬜⬜⬜⬜⬜

2. *Outer covering* MEERCODT ⬜⬜⬜⬜⬜⬜⬜⬜

3. *Converting mechanism* GEAVECLA ⬜⬜⬜⬜⬜⬜⬜⬜

4. *Genetic map* YOKAPRETY ⬜⬜⬜⬜⬜⬜⬜⬜⬜

5. *Future embryo* TOYSCBALST ⬜⬜⬜⬜⬜⬜⬜⬜⬜⬜

6. *Union result* GOTEYZ ⬜⬜⬜⬜⬜⬜

7. *From ectoderm* NETUCREDMOORE ⬜⬜⬜⬜⬜⬜⬜⬜⬜⬜⬜⬜⬜

8. *Embryonic tissue* CESHEMENYM ⬜⬜⬜⬜⬜⬜⬜⬜⬜⬜

9. *First draft* RORPUDMIMI ⬜⬜⬜⬜⬜⬜⬜⬜⬜⬜

10. *Avoid toxicity* EGRAOENTTS ⬜⬜⬜⬜⬜⬜⬜⬜⬜⬜

CHAPTER 4

1. *Nose bump* RACTIEGAL ⬜⬜⬜⬜⬜⬜⬜⬜⬜

2. *Gill time* CHIALRANB ⬜⬜⬜⬜⬜⬜⬜⬜⬜

3. *Disappearance act* KEECLM ⬜⬜⬜⬜⬜⬜

4. *Neck bone* DIHOY ⬜⬜⬜⬜⬜

5. *Sense button* DLAPSECO ⬜⬜⬜⬜⬜⬜⬜⬜

6. *Outer doughnut* RATELLA ⬜⬜⬜⬜⬜⬜⬜

7. *Open communication* NEEMBARM ⬜⬜⬜⬜⬜⬜⬜⬜

8. *Four evaginations* CPHOSUE ⬜⬜⬜⬜⬜⬜⬜

9. *Upper facial* SOOFNTNAARL ⬜⬜⬜⬜⬜⬜⬜⬜⬜⬜⬜

10. *Primitive landmark* MTOODEMUS ⬜⬜⬜⬜⬜⬜⬜⬜⬜

CHAPTER 5

1. *Tight tongue* AAGYOINSSKLOL ⬜⬜⬜⬜⬜⬜⬜⬜⬜⬜⬜⬜
2. *Parting tissues* LETCF ⬜⬜⬜⬜⬜
3. *From fourth* TEIPLIGOCT ⬜⬜⬜⬜⬜⬜⬜⬜⬜
4. *Stacked six* IESGLWLNS ⬜⬜⬜⬜⬜⬜⬜⬜
5. *Funny thing* AULVU ⬜⬜⬜⬜⬜
6. *Overgrowing base* OUPALC ⬜⬜⬜⬜⬜⬜
7. *Middle meeting* LESVHSE ⬜⬜⬜⬜⬜⬜⬜
8. *Roof parts* AALPLAT ⬜⬜⬜⬜⬜⬜⬜
9. *Initial tongue* RETMCUBUUL ⬜⬜⬜⬜⬜⬜⬜⬜⬜⬜
10. *In midline* AIPRM ⬜⬜⬜⬜⬜

CHAPTER 6

1. *Empty slot* OOAANDINT ⬜⬜⬜⬜⬜⬜⬜⬜
2. *Leftover cells* ZELSMAAS ⬜⬜⬜⬜⬜⬜⬜
3. *Twining trouble* NOIEGMIATN ⬜⬜⬜⬜⬜⬜⬜⬜⬜
4. *Primary shedders* STOSLAODNTOC ⬜⬜⬜⬜⬜⬜⬜⬜⬜⬜⬜
5. *Early form* IOMCEETND ⬜⬜⬜⬜⬜⬜⬜⬜
6. *Secretory surface* SMTEO ⬜⬜⬜⬜⬜
7. *Compressed layer* MMDIUNTREEI ⬜⬜⬜⬜⬜⬜⬜⬜⬜⬜
8. *Second draft* NUUCDSCEAEOS ⬜⬜⬜⬜⬜⬜⬜⬜⬜⬜
9. *Merry myth* YIFAR ⬜⬜⬜⬜⬜
10. *Accessory cusps* BEECLSTUR ⬜⬜⬜⬜⬜⬜⬜⬜

CHAPTER 7

1. *Cytoplasm spaces* VAUCLEOS ⬜⬜⬜⬜⬜⬜⬜
2. *Splitting up* SOMTIIS ⬜⬜⬜⬜⬜⬜

3. *Junction tie* DOSMMEOSE □□□□□□□□□

4. *Cell center* ULCELOUNS □□□□□□□□□

5. *Moving out* OSSEYTOXIC □□□□□□□□□□

6. *Breaking down* MESYSLOOS □□□□□□□□□

7. *Chromatin condenses* ROSHAEPP □□□□□□□□

8. *Two chromatids* TEMRONEECR □□□□□□□□□□

9. *Rough guys* SRIMBOOES □□□□□□□□□

10. *Major player* FEMSTOINNOLAT □□□□□□□□□□□□□

CHAPTER 8

1. *Mineral identification* PAAYTHRIODXYTE □□□□□□□□□□□□□□

2. *Nutrition canals* CIALNAULIC □□□□□□□□□

3. *Vessel wrapping* THELENDOMUI □□□□□□□□□□□

4. *Layered epithelium* EFADISTRTI □□□□□□□□□

5. *Hard rings* TONESSO □□□□□□□

6. *Making fibers* BIABSLFROT □□□□□□□□□

7. *Alien stuff* NIOMUMENG □□□□□□□□

8. *Replacement clocking* ORVENTUR □□□□□□□□

9. *Clot creation* TELLEPAST □□□□□□□□□

10. *Nerve communication* NYSASEP □□□□□□□

CHAPTER 9

1. *Unique tissue* TEZEKPAIRNADAIR □□□□□□□□□□□□□□□

2. *Waterproofing tactic* RAKTENI □□□□□□□

3. *Dark spots* LUGREANS □□□□□□□□

4. *Gum tufting* TIGPIPSLN □□□□□□□□□

5. *Blood group* ACALPRILY □□□□□□□□□

6. *Down deeper* BOSSAMUUC ☐☐☐☐☐☐☐☐☐

7. *Italy map* PHIRGAEOCG ☐☐☐☐☐☐☐☐☐☐

8. *Over bone* SMUMEPOCEIROTU ☐☐☐☐☐☐☐☐☐☐☐☐☐☐

9. *Tongue field* ZISPAEECLID ☐☐☐☐☐☐☐☐☐☐☐

10. *Dried up* KEPICRL ☐☐☐☐☐☐☐

CHAPTER 10

1. *Between layers* NALAMI ☐☐☐☐☐☐

2. *Facing tooth* LAVDENINGTOGI ☐☐☐☐☐☐☐☐☐☐☐☐☐

3. *Always young* JOUCTIANNL ☐☐☐☐☐☐☐☐☐☐

4. *Periodontal playground* LUULSCRA ☐☐☐☐☐☐☐☐

5. *Future measurement* VUCRRIECLA ☐☐☐☐☐☐☐☐☐☐

6. *Growing gums* HYSAPARLEPI ☐☐☐☐☐☐☐☐☐☐☐

7. *Long teeth* CORSEESIN ☐☐☐☐☐☐☐☐☐

8. *Sore gums* TIINVSGIGI ☐☐☐☐☐☐☐☐☐☐

9. *Deeper disease* KEOPCT ☐☐☐☐☐☐

10. *Continued infection* DIREPOONTIITS ☐☐☐☐☐☐☐☐☐☐☐☐☐

CHAPTER 11

1. *Group secretion* SANCIU ☐☐☐☐☐☐

2. *Gland masses* ELFSOLILC ☐☐☐☐☐☐☐☐☐

3. *Node depression* HUISL ☐☐☐☐☐

4. *Bigger grapes* PYHMDAPELONTYAH ☐☐☐☐☐☐☐☐☐☐☐☐☐☐☐

5. *Nasal projections* OCCHENA ☐☐☐☐☐☐☐

6. *Desert place* XOOERASMTI ☐☐☐☐☐☐☐☐☐☐

7. *Head spaces* RANSPALAA ☐☐☐☐☐☐☐☐☐

8. *Damp kisser* ILASAV ☐☐☐☐☐☐

9. *Making thyroxine* DOLICLO ☐☐☐☐☐☐☐

10. *Lymphoid masses* TALOLNSIR ☐☐☐☐☐☐☐☐☐

CHAPTER 12

1. *Breaking crystals* FABTCANRIO ☐☐☐☐☐☐☐☐☐☐

2. *Dark brushes* FUSTT ☐☐☐☐☐

3. *Rubbed out* BANRAISO ☐☐☐☐☐☐☐☐

4. *Faulty enamel* PDSSYILAA ☐☐☐☐☐☐☐☐☐

5. *Short tubules* NIESDSPL ☐☐☐☐☐☐☐☐

6. *Named layers* TRIESZU ☐☐☐☐☐☐☐

7. *Hardrock bands* AICTMBRINIO ☐☐☐☐☐☐☐☐☐☐☐

8. *Worn jewel* NOTATRITI ☐☐☐☐☐☐☐☐☐

9. *Interrod enamel* PRIIMTERICTSNA ☐☐☐☐☐☐☐☐☐☐☐☐☐☐

10. *Outer grooviness* KYMPERATIA ☐☐☐☐☐☐☐☐☐☐

CHAPTER 13

1. *Whole hole* MONFRAE ☐☐☐☐☐☐☐

2. *Disturbed apposition* TURCONO ☐☐☐☐☐☐☐

3. *Around middle* CUCPIRAUMPLL ☐☐☐☐☐☐☐☐☐☐☐☐

4. *First covering* NETMAL ☐☐☐☐☐☐

5. *Around tubes* BUTLERAPIUR ☐☐☐☐☐☐☐☐☐☐☐

6. *Tubule type* TNADELIN ☐☐☐☐☐☐☐☐

7. *Lateral complications* RAOSCECSY ☐☐☐☐☐☐☐☐☐

8. *Avoid ice* VEISHYPIERSNITTY ☐☐☐☐☐☐☐☐☐☐☐☐☐☐☐☐

9. *Named layers* BERNE ☐☐☐☐☐

10. *Inner pain* TULSPIPI ☐☐☐☐☐☐☐☐

CHAPTER 14

1. *Trouble scaling* PURSS ☐☐☐☐☐
2. *No cells* RACELALUL ☐☐☐☐☐☐☐☐☐
3. *Two kinds* NELMSECTICE ☐☐☐☐☐☐☐☐☐☐
4. *Dental nightmare* EUSUDENTOL ☐☐☐☐☐☐☐☐☐
5. *Bulk fibers* QUOIBLE ☐☐☐☐☐☐☐
6. *Extra extra* ISHTYMERCEPENSO ☐☐☐☐☐☐☐☐☐☐☐☐☐☐☐
7. *Probing junction* MEECLEMENTONA ☐☐☐☐☐☐☐☐☐☐☐☐☐
8. *Between roots* RACDILTERIUARN ☐☐☐☐☐☐☐☐☐☐☐☐☐☐
9. *Supporting team* TERIMOODPINU ☐☐☐☐☐☐☐☐☐☐☐☐
10. *Ninety degrees* YESHARPS ☐☐☐☐☐☐☐☐

CHAPTER 15

1. *Meeting place* TACONCT ☐☐☐☐☐☐☐
2. *Floss heaven* INOXTMERPRIAL ☐☐☐☐☐☐☐☐☐☐☐☐☐
3. *Bite me* SOONCLUIC ☐☐☐☐☐☐☐☐☐
4. *In orthodontics* LEPARM ☐☐☐☐☐☐
5. *Four squares* DANQTUARNS ☐☐☐☐☐☐☐☐☐☐
6. *Linear elevations* GRISED ☐☐☐☐☐☐
7. *Root caves* VITANESCOCI ☐☐☐☐☐☐☐☐☐☐☐
8. *Six slices* XSASENTT ☐☐☐☐☐☐☐☐
9. *More specific* HIRSTD ☐☐☐☐☐☐
10. *Talking points* AUSLNIVER ☐☐☐☐☐☐☐☐☐

CHAPTER 16

1. *Traumatic injury* NALVUISO ☐☐☐☐☐☐☐☐
2. *Back side* CUIMGLUN ☐☐☐☐☐☐☐☐

3. *Older term* DUCSPI ☐☐☐☐☐☐

4. *Cute space* STIEAMAD ☐☐☐☐☐☐☐☐

5. *Odd incisor* CHONTUSHINS ☐☐☐☐☐☐☐☐☐☐☐

6. *Getting depressed* SOAFSE ☐☐☐☐☐☐

7. *Canine retained* PIAMDCET ☐☐☐☐☐☐☐☐

8. *New ridge* SIACLIN ☐☐☐☐☐☐☐

9. *Even cuter* LOESMNAM ☐☐☐☐☐☐☐☐

10. *Extra something* EOSEDIMNS ☐☐☐☐☐☐☐☐☐

CHAPTER 17

1. *Older term* SPUDICIB ☐☐☐☐☐☐☐☐

2. *Maxillary special* QOEUBIL ☐☐☐☐☐☐☐

3. *Cute cusp* CLERIABAL ☐☐☐☐☐☐☐☐☐

4. *Angular distortion* LEDIARTOCAIN ☐☐☐☐☐☐☐☐☐☐☐☐

5. *Elongated depression* TULFGIN ☐☐☐☐☐☐☐

6. *Hidden areas* SHERCOTC ☐☐☐☐☐☐☐☐

7. *Odd molar* BUMLYRER ☐☐☐☐☐☐☐☐

8. *Deep grooves* UFINSO ☐☐☐☐☐☐

9. *Between roots* AURCFINOT ☐☐☐☐☐☐☐☐☐

10. *Three roots* TERICFRATUD ☐☐☐☐☐☐☐☐☐☐☐

CHAPTER 18

1. *Special spaces* MIPERAT ☐☐☐☐☐☐☐

2. *Prominent ridge* RIAVCECL ☐☐☐☐☐☐☐☐

3. *Large chamber* LUPP ☐☐☐☐

4. *Risky restorative* NORSH ☐☐☐☐☐

5. *Early childhood* SECAIR ☐☐☐☐☐☐

6. *Stained teeth* NAMTHYSS ☐☐☐☐☐☐☐☐

7. *Good start* MRIYPAR ☐☐☐☐☐☐☐

8. *Kid grinding* XIRSBUM ☐☐☐☐☐☐☐

9. *Worn tops* OARNTTITI ☐☐☐☐☐☐☐☐☐

10. *Whiter smile* EELANM ☐☐☐☐☐☐

CHAPTER 19

1. *Raising mandible* VEAOINLET ☐☐☐☐☐☐☐☐☐

2. *Inferior depression* CAARITLUR ☐☐☐☐☐☐☐☐☐

3. *Joint fluid* YNOILVSA ☐☐☐☐☐☐☐☐

4. *Side movement* TELLARA ☐☐☐☐☐☐☐

5. *Working muscles* MOICTASAITN ☐☐☐☐☐☐☐☐☐☐☐

6. *Sharper ridge* GLOPOSTEDIN ☐☐☐☐☐☐☐☐☐☐☐

7. *Partial dislocation* BUIUBLXATSON ☐☐☐☐☐☐☐☐☐☐☐☐

8. *Joint pain* SRIDDORE ☐☐☐☐☐☐☐☐

9. *Joint cover* LEAPSCU ☐☐☐☐☐☐☐

10. *Jaw backward* TROINRACTE ☐☐☐☐☐☐☐☐☐☐

CHAPTER 20

1. *Noisy occlusion* MRUIBXS ☐☐☐☐☐☐☐

2. *Mandible facial* TROSBSICE ☐☐☐☐☐☐☐☐☐

3. *Lateral curve* NOLSIW ☐☐☐☐☐☐

4. *Resting mandible* RLEANECAC ☐☐☐☐☐☐☐☐☐

5. *Smaller premolars* WEEYLA ☐☐☐☐☐☐

6. *Major disharmony* MRATAU ☐☐☐☐☐☐

7. *Habitually centric* OINCUCLSO ☐☐☐☐☐☐☐☐☐

8. *More women* ROIVEEBT ☐☐☐☐☐☐☐☐

9. *Horizontal overhang* JOEVETR ☐☐☐☐☐☐☐

10. *Occlusal classification* GALSNE ☐☐☐☐☐☐

UNIT I: REVIEW OF DENTAL STRUCTURES

Crossword

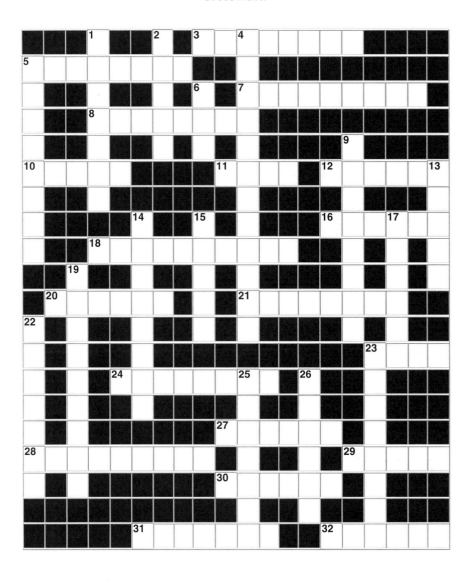

Across:

3 Vertical groove on midline of upper lip

5 Bony process or projection at anterior border of mandibular ramus

7 Small yellowish mucosa elevations resulting from misplaced sebaceous glands

8 Portion of maxilla or mandible that supports teeth

10 Nostrils of nose

11 Nasal region, external main feature (Do not blow it!)

12 Describes structures or facial surfaces of a tooth closest to inner cheek

16 Alveolar bone between two neighboring teeth, also called *interdental*

18 Part of the face that has many structures within it such as the lips and oral cavity

20 Hard inner crown layer of tooth overlying pulp

21 Socket of tooth

23 White ridge of raised keratinized epithelial tissue or linea on buccal mucosa

24 Lower jaw

27 Hard outer crown layer of tooth

28 Normal variation in bone growths on facial surface of maxillary alveolar process

29 Bony socket that contains eyeball and supporting structures

30 Space facing sulcular gingiva

31 Bony projection off posterior and superior border of mandibular ramus

32 Voice box in the midline of neck that is composed of cartilages

Down:

1 Opening from the pulp at the apex of the tooth

2 Keratinization where the teeth occlude

4 Facial region located both inferior to orbital region and lateral to nasal region

5 Outermost layer of the root of a tooth

6 Winglike cartilaginous structure laterally around the nares

9 Midline thickening of the upper lip

13 Tissue fluid that drains from surrounding region into lymphatic vessels

14 Small elevated structures of specialized mucosa on the tongue

15 Depression located where sulcus terminalis points backward toward pharynx

17 Nonencapsulated masses of lymphoid tissue

19 Darker appearance or zone of the lips compared with surrounding skin

22 Anteriors that are also the third teeth from the midline in each quadrant

23 Teeth type that includes incisors and canines located at the front of oral cavity

25 Describes structures or tooth surfaces closest to the tongue

26 Midline tissue fold between ventral surface of the tongue and floor of the mouth

Words to Find

Ala	Infraorbital	Nose	Submandibular
Angle	Labiomental	Orbit	Submental
Apex	Larynx	Parathyroid	Sulcus
Articulating	Lymph	Parotid	Symphysis
Buccal	Mandible	Philtrum	Temporomandibular
Commissure	Masseter	Proportions	Thyroid
Condyle	Mental	Ramus	Tubercle
Coronoid	Naris	Root	Vermilion
Frontal	Nasal	Sternocleidomastoid	Zygomatic
Hyoid	Nasolabial	Sublingual	

Word Search, Puzzle 1

```
L A R Y N X S K P R O P O R T I O N S I
S R D O G Z H L A T N O R F T O O R D R
I Y A I R E L C R E B U T S Y L W I A Y
S S E L O D I O R Y H T A R A P O L L D
Y S L A U Y H N O S E H Q L O T U A I E
H I Y T G B H P C U S P A A S B T O R S
P R D N E J I I M U Y I L A I I R U U B
M A N E N W T D B Y B A M D B Y S C L M
Y N O M B A J L N A L O N R H S L A Q A
S H C B M A I E L A D A O T I U B V L S
C J U O N N F O L I M A L M S I G A R S
C I G G G K S M E B R O M N O X T B V E
T Y L U E A T L U F I O R M B N E X B T
Z E A Z N N C S N L C D E O E U P P J E
L L V F K O U I U A A N N M P A C X A R
M D I O N O R O C M T S B A R M Y C Y R
A M U R T L I H P A A U A O M I E M A L
P I E A X Q M E L I S R T N J A N T U L
E T C Z E R A H A R T I C U L A T I N G
S N O I L I M R E V D T I B R O G P Z V
```

Words to Find

Alveolar	Foliate	Mucogingival	Raphe
Alveolus	Fordyce's	Mucosa	Retromolar
Anterior	Fornix	Nasopharynx	Submandibular
Caruncle	Fungiform	Oropharynx	Taste
Cecum	Gingiva	Parotid	Terminalis
Dorsal	Incisors	Periodontal	Tonsil
Exostoses	Labial	Permanent	Torus
Facial	Lingual	Posterior	Tuberosity
Fauces	Mastication	Premolars	Uvula
Faucial	Melanin	Primary	Ventral
Filiform	Molars	Pterygomandibular	Vestibules
Fimbriata	Mucobuccal	Pulp	

Word Search, Puzzle 2

```
T  S  R  O  S  I  C  N  I  F  P  R  I  M  A  R  Y  F  V  T
S  L  D  E  G  N  L  M  I  L  V  S  A  Q  R  R  R  O  E  O
R  H  A  G  L  A  O  M  R  E  A  S  U  O  W  A  A  L  N  N
A  N  O  V  I  C  B  I  S  O  O  U  I  L  L  L  P  I  T  S
L  Y  U  B  I  R  N  T  T  C  F  R  G  U  O  O  H  A  R  I
O  Y  A  L  I  G  I  U  U  A  E  I  B  N  U  E  E  T  A  L
M  L  T  A  A  B  N  M  R  T  C  I  L  X  I  V  V  E  L  S
E  X  T  I  U  C  L  I  N  A  D  I  W  I  S  L  U  L  I  O
R  A  N  L  S  A  C  A  G  N  C  N  T  U  F  A  J  L  A  L
P  T  E  Y  I  O  D  U  A  O  A  E  B  S  A  T  A  S  A  R
Z  S  N  C  R  O  R  M  B  S  C  M  C  W  A  N  X  T  A  M
F  R  U  E  R  A  O  E  O  O  A  U  E  U  I  M  N  L  R  Y
P  A  O  S  N  G  H  P  B  N  C  X  M  M  M  O  O  O  F  R
F  G  A  I  Y  A  H  P  D  U  O  U  R  U  D  M  F  O  P  M
F  L  I  R  R  A  M  I  O  S  T  E  M  O  O  I  R  A  F  E
W  A  E  N  R  E  B  R  T  R  T  S  I  R  G  D  R  O  A  L
F  T  U  Y  G  U  T  O  E  A  O  R  T  N  Y  O  R  P  C  A
P  A  N  C  L  I  S  S  S  P  E  E  U  C  T  N  U  E  I  N
O  X  T  A  E  E  V  T  O  P  R  F  E  I  I  L  N  F  A  I
T  O  R  U  S  S  E  A  T  P  H  S  D  X  P  I  J  H  L  N
```

UNIT II: DENTAL EMBRYOLOGY

Crossword, Puzzle 1

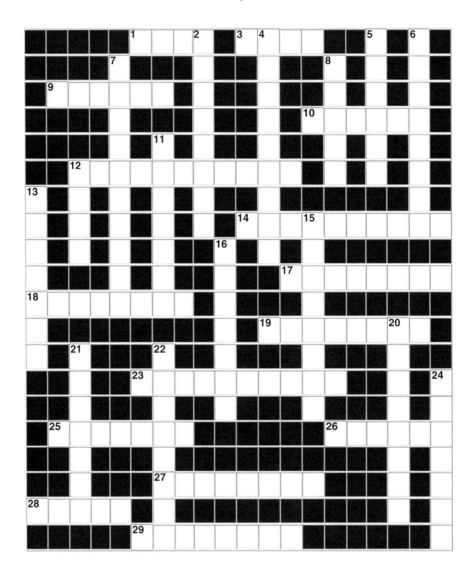

Across:

1   Circular plate of bilayered cells developed from the blastocyst

3   Depressions in the center of each nasal placode that evolve into the nasal cavities

9   Elimination of this structure between two adjacent swellings during fusion

10 Type of tube formed when neural folds meet and fuse superior to the neural groove

12 Cells that differentiate from preameloblasts forming enamel during amelogenesis

14 Form of a structure

17 Embryonic layer located between ectoderm and endoderm

18 Superior layer in the bilaminar disc

19 Areas of ectoderm found located at developing special sense organs on embryo

23 Embryonic disc with three distinct layers: ectoderm, mesoderm, and endoderm

25 Fused internal and inferior growth from paired medial nasal processes on inside of stomodeum

26 Tail end of a structure such as in the trilaminar embryonic disc

27 Primitive streak causes so that each half of disc mirrors the other half of the embryo

28 Structure of fetal period of prenatal development derived from enlarged embryo

29 Process during prenatal development when mitosis converts a zygote to a blastocyst

Down:

2   Head end of a structure such as in the trilaminar embryonic disc

4   Action of one group of cells on another leads to the establishment of developmental pathway in responding tissue

5   Structure derived from the implanted blastocyst

6   Posterior _____ develops from fourth branchial arches marking the development of future epiglottis

7   Developmental problems evident at birth are _____ malformations

8   Specialized group of cells developed from neuroectoderm that migrate from the neural folds

11 Paired cuboidal aggregates of cells differentiated from the mesoderm

12 Branchial apparatus includes branchial _____, branchial grooves and membranes, and pharyngeal pouches

13 Cleft lip is failure of fusion of maxillary processes with medial nasal _____

15 Processes that occur from the start of pregnancy to birth of the child

16 Membrane at the caudal end of the embryo that is the future anus

20 Layer in the trilaminar embryonic disc derived from the epiblast layer that lines stomodeum

21 Anterior portion of future digestive tract or primitive pharynx forming oropharynx

22 Embryonic membrane disintegrates bringing nasal and oral cavities into communication

24 Process occurring to embryo, placing the tissues in proper positions

Crossword, Puzzle 2

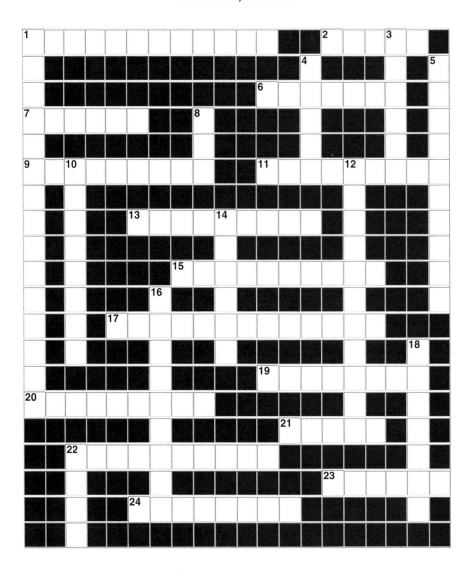

Across:

1 Groove that extends from medial corner of the eye to nasal cavity

2 Developmental disturbance due to failure of fusion of palatal shelves with primary palate/each other

6 Two processes derived from the maxillary processes during prenatal development

7 Portion of cervical loop that functions to shape root(s) inducing root dentin formation

9 Cementum matrix laid down by cementoblasts

11 Circular plate of bilayered cells developed from the blastocyst

13 Process by which action of one group of cells on another that leads to establishing the developmental pathway in the responding tissue

15 Layered formation of a firm or hard tissue such as cartilage, bone, enamel, dentin, or cementum

17 Process by which the sperm penetrates the ovum during preimplantation period

19 Photographic analysis of chromosomes

20 Primitive mouth appearing as shallow depression in embryonic surface

21 Cap or bell-shaped portion of tooth germ that produces enamel

22 Prenatal structure of trophoblast cells and inner cell mass that develop into embryo

23 Substance in connective tissue composed of intercellular substance and fibers or extracellular substance that is partially calcified and serves as a framework for later calcification

24 Layer in the trilaminar embryonic disc derived from hypoblast layer

Down:

1 Permanent teeth without primary predecessors, also known as *molars*.

3 Dental developmental disturbance in which adjacent tooth germs unite

4 Small, spherical enamel projection

5 Removal of hard tissue such as bone, enamel, dentin, or cementum

8 Second stage with growth of dental lamina into ectomesenchyme

10 Groups of epithelial cells of _____ in periodontal ligament (PDL) after disintegration of Hertwig's epithelial root sheath (HERS)

12 Abnormally small teeth

14 Pair of posterior swellings formed from both third and fourth branchial arches, which overgrow second branchial arches.

16 Dentin matrix laid down by apposition by the odontoblasts

18 Process of reproductive cell production that ensures correct number of chromosomes.

22 Fourth stage of odontogenesis in which differentiation occurs to its furthest extent.

Words to Find

Amniocentesis	Ectoderm	Induction	Primordium
Bilaminar	Embryo	Karyotype	Somites
Blastocyst	Endoderm	Maturation	Symmetry
Caudal	Epiblast	Meiosis	Teratogens
Cephalic	Fertilization	Mesoderm	Trilaminar
Cleavage	Fetus	Mitosis	Zygote
Cloacal	Folding	Morphology	
Congenital	Fusion	Neuroectoderm	
Disc	Hypoblast	Prenatal	

Word Search, Puzzle 1

```
Q F E V U D C L L S F D C L E A V A G E
A B P T X S F L M E S O D E R M S M L S
Q E I R S Y M M E T R Y B I H N R A I N
C C B I B L A S T O C Y S T E E T S O S
L T L L M I T O S I S G R G D I E I U W
O O A A W R C L V S J S O O N T T T E P
A D S M Y J A N I A E T T E N C E T R H
C E T I W D G S G T A C G E U F F D P Z
A R M N U B O D I R E N C D E P E Q R C
L M E A C I L M E O O O N C H I R J E R
M G C R E U O T R C I I P M Y D T K N O
J A B M F S Y U C N H K R O P S I U A E
F C T I X O E W M U U A I R O A L E T M
U E M U L N L A J H R R M P B B I N A B
S P D R R A Z D O Q I Y O H L X Z D L R
I H J H A A M Y I U Y O R O A S A O U Y
O A D G L Z T I G N U T D L S F T D H O
N L J I R D L I N O G Y I O T F I E Z T
K I U J S S V F O A T P U G C L O R Q B
B C Q T O C K O H N R E M Y L K N M X V
```

Words to Find

Apposition	Ectomesenchyme	Membrane	Preameloblasts
Bell	Fusion	Microdontia	Predentin
Bud	Gemination	Morphogenesis	Repolarization
Cementoblasts	Induction	Nonsuccedaneous	Resorption
Cementocytes	Initiation	Odontoblasts	Sheath
Cementoid	Macrodontia	Odontoclasts	Succedaneous
Dilaceration	Malassez	Organ	Supernumerary
Ectoderm	Matrix	Pearl	

Word Search, Puzzle 2

```
W C X O O X X L C E M E N T O C Y T E S
M M A L A S S E Z E N N N N S N S S V X
I B S F U S I O N I O O O I O T U K I E
C R E S Y G K A T I I I S I S O Y R O S
R Z X L P J R N T T E T A E F T O T O
O F P Q L B E A I A N A L N O A S S B L
D C C L M D N S I E Z B A E M N A X R N
O E Z E E I O T G I O D V C H L W A A S
N M M R M P I O R L E E N T B F E G O U
T E P E P N H A E C Z O A O M P R I D P
I N G A I P L M C G I E T M A O R N O E
A T D D R O A U Q T H N K E C C E D N R
R O U O P E S J A S O O B S R E S U T N
O B M E R N L R H D E H M E O M O C O U
E L R P O Q E S O T Y Q R N D E R T C M
K A W N E C E B M Q N D M C O N P I L E
I S R C A E C T O D E R M H N T T O A R
R T U L N E Q L J M D F B Y T O I N S A
A S I S D P B I O Y P C U M I I O F T R
C D J A S U W R V E E R T E A D N H S Y
```

UNIT III: DENTAL HISTOLOGY

Crossword, Puzzle 1

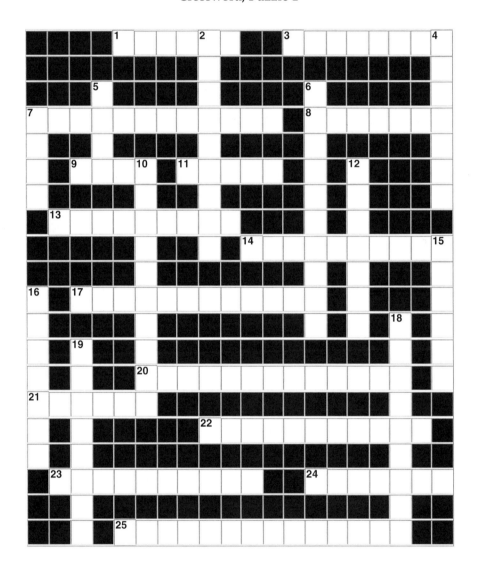

Across:

1 Group of organs functioning together

3 Closely apposed sheets of bone tissue in compact bone

7 Organelles associated with manufacture of adenosine triphosphate

8 Largest, densest, and most conspicuous organelle in the cell

9 Smallest unit of organization in the body

11 Somewhat independent body part that performs a specific function(s)

13 Chief nucleoprotein in the nondividing nucleoplasm

14 White blood cell (WBC) that increases in numbers during an immune response

17 The three-dimensional system of support within the cell

20 Type of intermediate filament with major role in intercellular junctions

21 Structure formed by cell groups with similar characteristics of shape and function.

22 Immature connective tissue formed during initial repair

23 Filamentous daughter chromosomes joined at a centromere during cell division

24 Specialized connective tissue composed of fat, little matrix, and adipocytes

25 Along with calcium, main inorganic crystal in enamel, bone, dentin, and cementum

Down:

2 Superficial layers of skin

4 Type of protein fiber in connective tissue composed of microfilaments

5 Rigid connective tissue

6 Metabolically inert substances or transient structures within the cell

7 WBC similar to basophil that is also involved in allergic responses

10 Second most common WBC in the blood

12 Portion of cell division resulting in two daughter cells identical to the parent cell

15 Small space that surrounds chondrocyte or osteocyte

16 Type of intermediate protein filament found in calloused epithelial tissues consisting of an opaque waterproof substance

18 Intercellular junction between cells

19 WBC that contains granules of histamine and heparin

Crossword, Puzzle 2

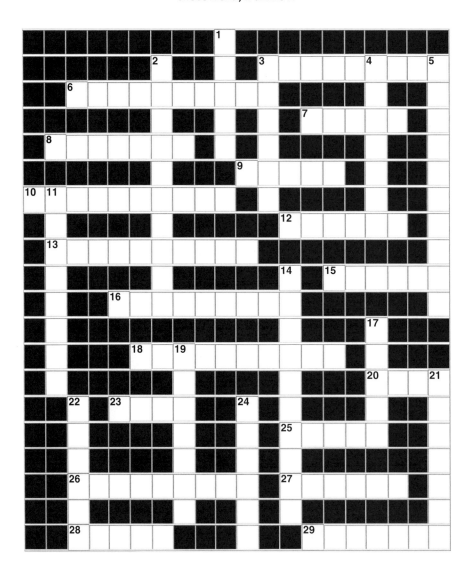

Across:

3 Tissue deep to oral mucosa composed of loose connective tissue

6 Joined matrix pieces forming lattice in cancellous bone

7 Tissue fluid that drains from the surrounding region into lymphatic vessels

8 Initially formed bone matrix

9 Central opening where saliva is deposited after being produced by secretory cells

10 Mature osteoblasts entrapped in bone matrix

12 Cells in respiratory mucosa that produce mucus to keep mucosa moist

13 Network of vessels that collect and transport lymph, linking body's lymph nodes

15 Hard tooth tissue loss resulting from demineralization due to acid produced by cariogenic bacteria

16 Blood cell fragments that function in clotting mechanism

18 Dense connective tissue layer on outer portion of bone

20 Extensions or ridges of the epithelium into connective tissue when viewing a histological section

23 Passageway that allows glandular secretion to be emptied directly into location where it is used

25 Large inner portions of certain glands

26 Dense connective tissue in dermis and lamina propria

27 Secretion from salivary glands that lubricates and cleanses oral cavity

28 Bundle of neural processes outside the central nervous system

29 Localized macules of pigmentation

Down:

1 Depression on one side of the lymph node

2 Grooves associated with lines of Retzius in enamel

3 Connective tissue that divides inner portion of certain glands

4 Connective tissue that surrounds outer portion of entire gland or lesion

5 Cells that differentiate from preameloblasts forming enamel during amelogenesis

11 Epithelium that stands away from the tooth, creating a gingival sulcus

14 Cells that function in resorption of bone

17 Nostril of nose

19 Incremental lines of _____ in histological preparations of mature enamel

21 Hard tooth tissue loss through chemical means not involving bacteria

22 Functional cellular component of the nervous system

24 Extracellular substance partially calcified, serving as framework for later calcification

Crossword, Puzzle 3

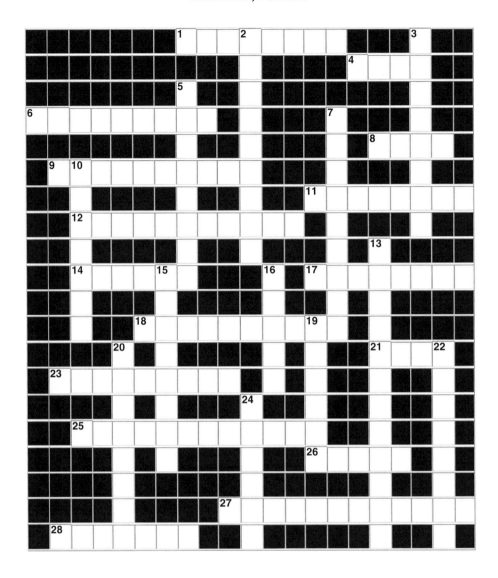

Across:

1 Inflammation of pulp

4 Soft innermost connective tissue in the crown and root

6 Hard tooth tissue loss by mastication or parafunctional habits

8 Crystalline structural unit of enamel that gives teeth the bright white

9 Layered formation of firm or hard tissue such as enamel, dentin, or cementum

11 Surrounds the teeth for support and attaches the teeth to the alveoli

12 Incremental lines or bands of von Ebner in mature dentin

14 Opening or foramen from the pulp at apex

17 Socket of tooth

18 Cancellous bone located between alveolar bone proper and plates of cortical bone

21 Imbrication lines in dentin demonstrating disturbance in body metabolism

23 Extra openings located on the lateral portions of the roots

25 Apposition of enamel matrix by ameloblasts

26 Microscopic enamel feature of small dark brushes with bases near the dentinoenamel junction (DEJ)

27 Layer of dentin around the outer pulpal wall

28 Portion of the tooth that contains the mass of pulp

Down:

2 Dentin matrix laid down by apposition by the odontoblasts

3 Microscopic enamel feature of short dentinal tubules near the DEJ

5 Plates of compact bone on the facial and lingual surfaces of the alveolar bone

7 Portion of the pulp located in the root area of the tooth

10 Dentin formed in a tooth before the completion of the apical foramen

13 Supporting hard/soft dental tissues between and including portions of the tooth and the alveolar bone

15 Hard tooth tissue loss by friction from toothbrushing and/or toothpaste

16 There is _____ within dentinal tubule in dentin

19 Smooth, stained microscopic lines in cartilage, bone, or cementum due to apposition

20 Outermost layer of the root of a tooth

22 Accentuated incremental line of Retzius or contour line of Owen from birth process

24 Hard inner layer of the crown of a tooth overlying pulp

Words to Find

Cell	Endocytosis	Microfilaments	Prophase
Centromere	Exocytosis	Microtubules	Ribosomes
Centrosome	Hemidesmosome	Mitochondria	System
Chromatids	Histology	Mitosis	Telophase
Chromatin	Inclusions	Nucleolus	Tissue
Chromosomes	Interphase	Nucleoplasm	Tonofilaments
Cytoplasm	Keratin	Nucleus	Vacuoles
Cytoskeleton	Lysosomes	Organ	
Desmosome	Metaphase	Phagocytosis	

Word Search, Puzzle 1

```
M I M E K W Q Q P H A G O C Y T O S I S
I J E X K U N W E E M S S S S S S E A A
T G T D B E U U S S I E I D S T S E I E
O D A I I K S A A S M S I U N A Q R M S
S M P K K S H L O O O T L E H S D O E M
I M H L I P P T S T A O M P E N S L S J
S J A T O O Y O Y M E A O M O O O A E S
M I S L T C M C O L L R O H R U L M T N
I N E Y O O O R C I P S C T C P O N I S
C T C X R D H U F Y O O N A O S E T N V
R E E H N C N O X M T E V E O M A O W E
O R C E P H R G S I C O L M A R I L R C
T P I C F C I E M N U C S L E S L E T H
U H G B I N D S A U U E I K U L M N Z R
B A S M O I U G T N D F I L E O S S T O
U S M S M S R C B O O L C C R L F Y O M
L E R E W O O M L N L N R T H P E S A A
E V H O O Q Z M O E I O N M B N H T D T
S D D Z D I Q T E C U E G R T H J E O I
L Y S O S O M E S S C S X Y Z N V M O N
```

Words to Find

Adipose
Appositional
Basophil
Bone
Canaliculi
Cartilage
Chondroblasts
Chondrocytes

Collagen
Dermis
Elastic
Endosteum
Endothelium
Eosinophil
Epidermis
Epithelium

Fibroblast
Granulation
Haversian
Hemidesmosomes
Hydroxyapatite
Immunogen
Immunoglobulin
Interstitial

Keratin
Lacuna
Lamellae
Lymphocyte
Macrophage
Mast

Word Search, Puzzle 2

```
N  E  S  J  X  J  V  B  O  N  E  C  A  R  T  I  L  A  G  E
M  A  S  T  E  P  I  T  H  E  L  I  U  M  L  A  C  U  N  A
U  J  E  I  J  C  B  D  L  M  X  B  D  R  O  Z  T  Z  I  C
W  I  L  M  J  H  E  I  U  L  A  M  E  L  L  A  E  L  F  W
I  J  A  M  O  O  I  M  M  U  N  O  G  L  O  B  U  L  I  N
H  Z  S  U  E  N  Q  K  V  M  M  E  P  I  D  E  R  M  I  S
I  C  T  N  A  D  D  E  R  M  I  S  D  R  O  K  X  Y  G  H
T  L  I  O  P  R  C  B  F  O  F  I  B  R  O  B  L  A  S  T
G  D  C  G  P  O  I  I  F  A  M  A  C  R  O  P  H  A  G  E
G  B  G  E  O  C  H  E  M  I  D  E  S  M  O  S  O  M  E  S
E  B  R  N  S  Y  Q  I  W  E  N  D  O  T  H  E  L  I  U  M
O  U  A  H  I  T  W  C  H  O  N  D  R  O  B  L  A  S  T  S
S  B  N  A  T  E  Q  C  P  V  A  J  C  O  L  L  A  G  E  N
I  A  U  V  I  S  J  A  D  I  P  O  S  E  Z  S  V  P  U  C
N  S  L  E  O  Y  G  J  D  S  D  D  R  K  E  R  A  T  I  N
O  O  A  R  N  Q  E  W  U  F  L  Y  M  P  H  O  C  Y  T  E
P  P  T  S  A  W  Z  S  I  N  T  E  R  S  T  I  T  I  A  L
H  H  I  I  L  K  C  U  O  B  I  E  N  D  O  S  T  E  U  M
I  I  O  A  R  F  H  Y  D  R  O  X  Y  A  P  A  T  I  T  E
L  L  N  N  W  J  Q  B  B  I  C  A  N  A  L  I  C  U  L  I
```

Words to Find

Endochondral
Intramembranous
Matrix
Monocyte
Nerve
Neuron
Neutrophil

Odontoclast
Ossification
Osteoblasts
Osteoclast
Osteocytes
Osteoid
Osteons

Papillary
Perichondrium
Periosteum
Plasma
Platelets
Rete
Reticular

Squames
Submucosa
Synapse
Tonofilaments
Trabeculae

Word Search, Puzzle 3

U	S	P	L	A	S	M	A	E	L	L	I	C	O	I	O	H	X	L	Z
B	U	T	F	Z	M	F	W	P	Y	R	X	F	Z	A	T	C	D	N	L
J	B	O	Y	Y	W	N	D	L	H	W	F	J	R	S	T	I	O	A	X
I	M	N	R	V	S	Y	N	A	P	S	E	F	A	H	O	I	R	S	M
V	U	O	E	F	K	F	O	T	J	I	W	L	O	E	T	D	K	U	B
P	C	F	T	L	I	B	X	E	S	H	C	T	T	A	N	U	E	A	K
L	O	I	I	Z	N	S	O	L	D	O	W	S	C	O	A	T	W	B	U
T	S	L	C	G	T	P	F	E	E	I	O	I	H	W	S	V	T	P	Z
L	A	A	U	V	R	G	W	T	E	P	F	C	H	O	O	S	F	E	G
B	C	M	L	O	A	S	S	S	C	I	O	S	I	E	A	E	P	R	X
L	T	E	A	S	M	O	P	V	S	D	C	R	T	L	V	O	A	I	N
E	R	N	R	T	E	N	L	S	N	K	E	Y	C	R	N	S	P	C	E
W	A	T	G	E	M	B	O	E	R	P	C	O	E	O	Z	T	I	H	U
O	B	S	S	O	B	D	R	I	D	O	T	N	Z	O	F	E	L	O	T
N	E	X	Q	B	R	R	G	X	N	N	C	W	M	S	B	O	L	N	R
E	C	K	U	L	A	P	P	O	O	M	V	K	A	T	V	C	A	D	O
U	U	B	A	A	N	K	M	D	A	V	E	C	T	E	K	Y	R	R	P
R	L	R	M	S	O	M	O	D	J	T	P	E	R	O	G	T	Y	I	H
O	A	J	E	T	U	N	K	W	E	A	J	S	I	N	K	E	W	U	I
N	E	T	S	S	S	F	K	R	I	C	U	H	X	S	B	S	X	M	L

Words to Find

Afferent	Germinal	Lobes	Periodontitis
Capsule	Gingivitis	Lobules	Prickle
Colloid	Goblet	Lumen	Recession
Dentogingival	Goiter	Lymph	Stippling
Duct	Granulation	Masticatory	Sulcular
Efferent	Hilus	Melanin	Sulcus
Endocrine	Hyperkeratinized	Mucogingival	Taste
Exocrine	Junctional	Mucoperiosteum	
Fibroblast	Keratin	Mucosa	
Follicles	Keratohyaline	Nodes	

Word Search, Puzzle 4

```
N  O  D  E  S  E  G  V  K  Y  Q  K  A  O  S  U  L  C  U  S
A  P  C  K  O  N  P  E  H  K  A  U  R  F  E  L  E  I  T  P
H  R  O  H  D  D  M  Z  R  G  E  E  S  N  F  N  Y  S  Y  T
A  I  L  H  K  O  U  U  D  M  T  R  I  L  I  E  A  M  C  D
E  C  L  Z  L  C  H  D  C  I  I  R  A  L  O  L  R  U  P  G
T  K  O  U  I  R  Y  E  O  O  C  N  A  T  B  B  D  E  N  H
A  L  I  T  S  I  P  G  G  O  P  Y  A  O  I  S  E  I  N  N
P  E  D  D  T  N  E  Y  X  O  H  E  R  L  E  N  L  S  O  T
E  S  W  E  A  E  R  E  E  O  B  B  R  L  M  P  B  I  Z  L
R  E  M  N  S  M  K  Z  T  A  I  L  C  I  P  G  S  S  A  N
I  G  A  T  T  U  E  A  M  F  T  I  E  I  O  S  T  V  O  S
O  I  S  O  E  D  R  L  P  S  L  E  T  T  E  S  I  I  E  Z
D  N  T  G  I  E  A  V  A  L  U  S  Z  C  N  G  T  L  W  A
O  G  I  I  K  C  T  V  O  N  I  L  E  L  N  A  U  E  S  V
N  I  C  N  E  A  I  F  X  G  I  R  C  I  L  B  Z  O  U  V
T  V  A  G  X  P  N  I  A  J  A  N  G  U  O  A  C  L  Y  M
I  I  T  I  V  S  I  M  O  M  J  O  N  L  L  U  P  U  U  N
T  T  O  V  F  U  Z  S  H  N  C  A  M  W  M  A  I  M  Z  L
I  I  R  A  D  L  E  P  B  U  R  M  E  F  F  E  R  E  N  T
S  S  Y  L  X  E  D  Z  M  G  J  U  N  C  T  I  O  N  A  L
```

Words to Find

Abfraction	Erosion	Parathyroid	Sinusitis
Abrasion	Lymphadenopathy	Perikymata	Thyroglossal
Ameloblast	Lymphatics	Ranula	Thyroid
Amelogenesis	Mucocele	Retzius	Thyroxine
Attrition	Mucoserous	Saliva	Tonsils
Caries	Myoepithelial	Secretory	Trabeculae
Demilune	Naris	Septum	Xerostomia

Word Search, Puzzle 5

```
I  B  W  S  T  H  Y  R  O  X  I  N  E  T  T  P  E  Z  P  B
S  A  B  F  R  A  C  T  I  O  N  N  K  F  S  K  Z  E  S  S
L  C  A  R  I  E  S  I  L  H  O  G  X  Z  V  I  A  U  I  A
P  A  R  A  T  H  Y  R  O  I  D  Y  E  U  Y  L  O  S  T  T
F  G  Y  L  S  I  N  U  S  I  T  I  S  H  U  R  E  A  S  N
G  D  Y  W  H  G  I  A  M  P  S  K  T  C  E  N  M  A  O  W
Y  E  D  M  U  U  R  X  L  R  N  A  E  S  E  Y  L  I  A  S
M  M  S  S  U  B  U  M  E  Y  P  B  O  G  K  B  T  D  C  D
U  I  A  E  A  J  C  Y  R  O  A  C  O  I  O  I  S  I  I  S
C  L  L  P  N  Z  W  O  N  R  U  L  R  L  R  V  T  O  U  N
O  U  I  T  I  W  T  E  T  M  E  E  E  T  D  A  R  I  O  C
C  N  V  U  U  E  D  P  E  M  P  M  T  F  H  Y  Z  I  D  L
E  E  A  M  R  A  Q  I  A  U  A  A  R  P  H  T  S  K  Q  F
L  H  T  C  H  U  R  T  Z  U  B  P  M  T  E  O  W  M  M  X
E  G  E  P  Y  G  A  H  R  F  R  Y  U  R  R  U  Q  I  G  W
P  S  M  F  Z  X  N  E  O  Y  L  W  G  E  R  G  D  A  N  T
X  Y  U  B  Z  A  U  L  E  F  X  E  R  O  S  T  O  M  I  A
L  K  N  K  S  F  L  I  C  Q  L  L  E  T  O  N  S  I  L  S
I  E  U  V  W  F  A  A  T  H  Y  R  O  G  L  O  S  S  A  L
P  H  T  B  F  V  N  L  N  A  R  I  S  B  F  W  H  S  U  Q
```

Words to Find

Accessory	Cementoid	Imbrication	Principal
Alveolus	Cementum	Interglobular	Pulp
Apical	Chamber	Intertubular	Pulpitis
Apposition	Circumpulpal	Mantle	Radicular
Arrest	Dentin	Neonatal	Secondary
Attrition	Dentinogenesis	Odontoblasts	Stones
Canaliculi	Edentulous	Owen	Tertiary
Cementicles	Fluid	Periodontium	Trabecular
Cementoblasts	Globular	Peritubular	Tubules
Cementocytes	Hypercementosis	Predentin	
Cementogenesis	Hypersensitivity	Primary	

Word Search, Puzzle 6

```
A T T A T Q M P N T G K O I B S A D C C
R E U L C P A U E R D A W M P T T B E H
R R B V E R N L O A E P E B R O T U M A
E T U E M I T P N B N I N R I N R B E M
S I L O E N L I A E T C H I M E I H N B
T A E L N C E T T C I A Y C A S T Z T E
C R S U T I C I A U N L P A R H I C U R
E Y P S O P E S L L O I E T Y Y O E M C
M P E C I A M E I A G N R I O P N M P E
E E R I D L E V N R E T S O D E K E R M
N R I R K C N E T Z N E E N O C A N E E
T I O C S A T D E R E R N A N E P T D N
I T D U E N O E R A S G S C T M P O E T
C U O M C A G N T D I L I C O E O C N O
L B N P O L E T U I S O T E B N S Y T B
E U T U N I N U B C F B I S L T I T I L
S L I L D C E L U U L U V S A O T E N A
U A U P A U S O L L U L I O S S I S W S
I R M A R L I U A A I A T R T I O Q R T
Y Q X L Y I S S R R D R Y Y S S N E Q S
```

Crossword, Puzzle 1

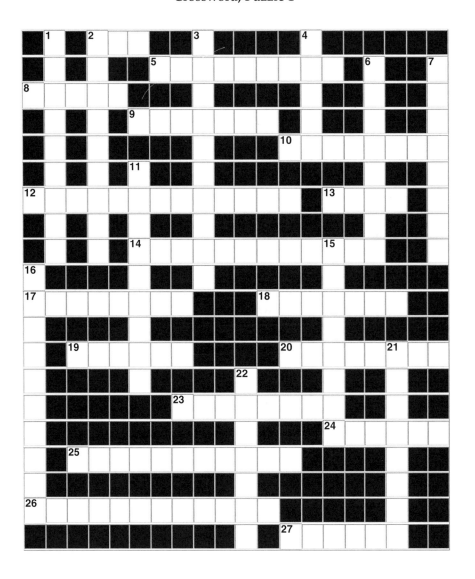

Across:

2 Small lateral incisor or third molar crown from partial microdontia

5 Natural teeth in the jaw consisting of both/either primary and permanent

8 Mythological creature, who at night takes children's shed primary teeth from under their pillows, leaving cold hard cash

9 Crest of curvature or greatest elevation of the tooth crown, either incisocervically or occlusocervically

10 Rounded enamel extensions on incisal ridge as noted from labial/lingual of anteriors

12 Tooth designation system using a two-digit code

13 Imaginary line representing long axis line of a tooth that bisects the cervical line

14 Crown or root(s) showing angular distortion

17 Rounded raised borders or ridges on mesial and distal portions of lingual surface of anteriors and occlusal table of posteriors

18 Older dental term for canines—thanks to our tail-wagging friends

19 Surface of a tooth closest to midline

20 Masticatory surface of posteriors

23 Vertically oriented and labially placed bony ridge of alveolar bone noted in jaws, especially in maxilla near canine

24 Surface of tooth farthest away from midline

25 Indentations on surface of the root(s)

26 Secondary groove on lingual surface of anteriors and occlusal table on posteriors

27 Division of a crown surface or root into three portions: crown horizontally and vertically and root horizontally

Down:

1 Division of each dental arch into two parts, with four quadrants for entire oral cavity

2 Second dentition

3 Portion of root covered by cementum

4 Shallow, wide depressions on lingual surface of anteriors or occlusal table of posteriors

6 Complete displacement of the tooth from the socket due to extensive trauma

7 Open contact existing between maxillary central incisors

11 Absence of a single tooth or multiple teeth due to lack of initiation

15 Unerupted/partially erupted tooth positioned against another tooth, bone, or even soft tissue

16 Spaces formed from the curvatures where two teeth in the same arch contact

21 Division of each dental arch into three portions based on midline

22 Linear elevation or ridge on incisal/masticatory surface of newly erupted incisors

Crossword, Puzzle 2

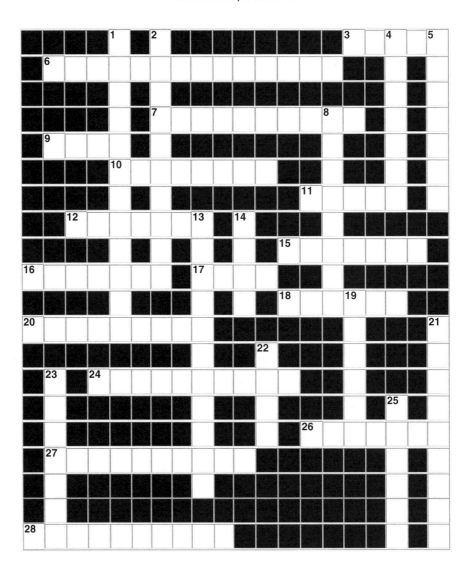

Across:

3 Situation in which entire posterior quadrant functions during lateral occlusion

6 Movements of the mandible that are not within the normal motions

7 Moving lower jaw forward

9 The _____ of the temporomandibular joint located between the temporal bone and mandibular condyle

10 Ridge running mesiodistally in the cervical one third of the buccal crown surface on the entire primary dentition and permanent molars

11 Natural movement of all of the teeth over time toward the midline of the oral cavity

12 Parafunctional habit of grinding teeth that sounds like a jet taking off

15 First dentition present, also known as *deciduous dentition*

16 Side to which the mandible has been moved during lateral occlusion

17 Type of terminal plane or _____ relationship with primary mandibular second molar mesial to the maxillary molar

18 Space created when primary molars are shed to make room for smaller mesiodistal permanent premolars

20 Other side of the arch from working side during lateral occlusion

24 Usually shows a rather prominent mandible and possibly a normal or even retrusive maxilla or concave profile

26 End point of closure of the mandible with it in its most retruded position

27 Lowering of lower jaw

28 Moving lower jaw backward

Down:

1 Failure to have overall ideal form to the dentition while in centric occlusion

2 Cusps that function during centric occlusion, including lingual cusps of maxillary posteriors, buccal cusps of mandibular posteriors, and incisal edges of mandibular anteriors

4 Maxillary dental arch facially overhangs the mandibular arch

5 Spaces between certain primary teeth

8 Situation in which the maxillary incisors also overlap the mandibular incisors

13 Facial profile in centric occlusion with slightly protruded jaws, giving the facial outline a relatively flat appearance or straight profile

14 If imaginary planes are placed on the masticatory surfaces of each dental arch, the maxillary arch is convex occlusally and the mandibular arch is concave

19 Concave curve results when a frontal section is taken through each set of both maxillary and mandibular molars—the first, second, and third molars

21 Parafunctional habit with teeth held in centric occlusion for long periods without a break into interocclusal clearance

22 Situation in which the canine is the only tooth in function during lateral occlusion

23 Bony projection off posterior and superior borders of the mandibular ramus

25 Occlusal _____ to periodontium resulting from occlusal disharmony

Words to Find

Anatomical	Cusp	Interproximal	Permanent
Axis	Deciduous	Masticatory	Primary
Cementoenamel	Dentition	Mesial	Proximal
Clinical	Distal	Midline	Quadrants
Concavities	Embrasures	Occlusal	Sextants
Contact	Incisal	Occlusion	Thirds
Contour	International	Palmar	Universal

Word Search, Puzzle 1

```
A  I  A  J  G  I  N  T  E  R  P  R  O  X  I  M  A  L  O  Q
T  H  I  R  D  S  T  L  T  L  R  V  F  L  Y  R  V  S  B  L
P  K  L  N  B  C  F  N  T  M  X  U  A  L  U  C  T  H  E  L
N  S  O  Z  A  A  E  G  Y  D  A  I  O  O  T  N  A  M  B  L
I  F  S  T  K  N  V  W  M  C  S  S  T  C  A  C  A  X  A  J
C  S  N  Z  A  A  U  E  O  E  O  N  T  T  C  N  K  N  I  L
T  O  V  M  B  T  N  T  M  K  O  N  X  I  E  L  O  X  A  S
C  C  R  P  S  O  I  G  E  C  V  E  C  O  C  I  U  M  L  C
H  E  U  Q  K  M  V  S  J  N  S  O  T  A  T  A  I  S  Y  E
P  N  W  S  K  I  E  D  J  Q  D  N  C  A  V  X  T  Q  A  L
L  R  L  R  P  C  R  B  U  E  E  I  N  C  O  I  N  O  A  L
W  V  I  E  R  A  S  Q  K  M  M  R  S  R  L  B  T  C  R  S
Z  C  N  M  D  L  A  U  E  R  E  B  P  T  C  U  I  I  U  Y
B  J  C  V  A  H  L  C  C  T  M  P  R  V  A  N  S  O  E  R
K  M  I  F  X  R  F  K  N  P  F  C  Y  A  I  L  U  I  E  S
Q  A  S  F  U  V  Y  I  A  I  Z  S  V  L  S  D  U  M  O  I
Z  W  A  U  X  O  N  R  J  M  S  J  C  Q  I  U  L  E  E  N
O  M  L  Q  U  A  D  R  A  N  T  S  Z  C  F  A  R  K  D  T
X  W  D  E  N  T  I  T  I  O  N  D  E  K  P  Q  Z  E  D  D
O  H  M  I  D  L  I  N  E  J  H  D  T  W  N  U  Q  X  S  P
```

Words to Find

Anodontia	Cuspids	Furcation	Peg
Avulsion	Dentigerous	Impacted	Supernumerary
Bicuspid	Diastema	Mamelons	Supplemental
Bifurcated	Dilaceration	Marginal	Transverse
Carabelli	Eminence	Mesiodens	Triangular
Central	Flutting	Mulberry	Trifurcated
Cingulum	Fossa	Multirooted	Tubercles

Word Search, Puzzle 2

```
P K A C B B I F U R C A T E D E U F F M
U O A I B T O S T Y E N L W D T D X R D
S I Z N N B I J U S W A U E D I O A E A
F M C G K A D M R P T S T D P Y L T A Q
L P J U T G K E A N E O N S Q U A S Y H
U A K L L Z V I E I O R U P G C S G E F
T C W U Y S T M G R S C N N R O R M F V
T T S M N N E L I L I K A U F O V F X E
I E U A O L H T L B H I F D M F X A R I
N D R D P W L Q D U R I Z I Z E X I Y Q
G T O P D U Y A E T R D X L Z I R G Q N
R N U R M F B T N T P C M A M S H A P P
A S M M E U K U T D E A A C P E A I R S
V C U A S R N B I I G R R E N M V C F Y
A U L M I C D E G A S A G R G I U E J L
P S B E O A H R E S L B I A O N L N X C
P P E L D T L C R T Z E N T D E S T D C
X I R O E I C L O E X L A I P N I R D O
I D R N N O B E U M K L L O S C O A D Y
U S Y S S N O S S A B I P N T E N L V X
```

Words to Find

Abfraction	Deviation	Overjet	Step
Articular	Disc	Parafunctional	Subluxation
Balancing	Drift	Premature	Supporting
Bruxism	Elevation	Primary	Synovial
Capsule	Group	Primate	Temporomandibular
Centric	Interocclusal	Prognathic	Terminal
Cervical	Leeway	Protrusion	Trauma
Clenching	Malocclusion	Retraction	Wilson
Condyle	Mesognathic	Retrognathic	Working
Crossbite	Occlusion	Rise	
Depression	Overbite	Spee	

Word Search, Puzzle 3

```
A  U  F  P  R  I  M  A  T  E  R  E  T  R  A  C  T  I  O  N
R  I  N  T  E  R  O  C  C  L  U  S  A  L  W  I  L  S  O  N
T  O  N  T  E  M  P  O  R  O  M  A  N  D  I  B  U  L  A  R
I  P  G  X  E  L  E  V  A  T  I  O  N  P  R  I  M  A  R  Y
C  O  N  D  Y  L  E  M  A  L  O  C  C  L  U  S  I  O  N  J
U  S  P  M  D  S  U  B  L  U  X  A  T  I  O  N  R  I  S  E
L  P  W  O  R  K  I  N  G  B  P  R  O  G  N  A  T  H  I  C
A  W  R  X  M  E  S  O  G  N  A  T  H  I  C  D  R  I  F  T
R  R  A  E  V  V  C  E  I  U  P  M  T  E  R  M  I  N  A  L
H  C  E  O  M  L  E  E  W  A  Y  D  E  V  I  A  T  I  O  N
D  L  P  T  M  A  P  A  R  A  F  U  N  C  T  I  O  N  A  L
E  E  B  R  R  X  T  T  O  V  E  R  B  I  T  E  S  T  E  P
P  N  A  S  O  O  Z  U  C  R  O  S  S  B  I  T  E  O  T  J
R  C  L  B  C  T  G  Q  R  T  F  O  C  C  L  U  S  I  O  N
E  H  A  R  T  E  R  N  C  E  R  V  I  C  A  L  S  P  E  E
S  I  N  U  R  G  N  U  A  V  A  B  F  R  A  C  T  I  O  N
S  N  C  X  A  R  D  T  S  T  S  U  P  P  O  R  T  I  N  G
I  G  I  I  U  O  I  X  R  I  H  H  S  Y  N  O  V  I  A  L
O  H  N  S  M  U  S  D  Y  I  O  I  X  O  V  E  R  J  E  T
N  W  G  M  A  P  C  Q  L  I  C  N  C  C  A  P  S  U  L  E
```

Guidelines
for Tooth
Drawing

Introduction

Tooth-drawing assignments emphasize fundamental principles in tooth design, which later have direct practical application in clinical coursework of a dental professional. Initial drawings are most likely to be the student's first attempts at capturing any tooth likeness; they will certainly encourage accuracy and discernment of the teeth and hopefully facilitate the recognition of tooth details. *Artistic inclinations are not really needed with these basic technical drawings.*

It is important to also note that these drawings are only two-dimensional and are somewhat limited to fundamental outlines and proportions. However, they will serve to help create mental pictures of teeth in their ideal or composite state. Remember that real specimens in patients' mouths vary considerably.

Activity Steps

1. Locate the two, blank gridded worksheets in the workbook. Any additional gridded worksheets needed can be easily copied for the correct spacing of the grid needed. Correctly label the worksheet at the bottom of the page with the tooth that will be drawn as shown in the smaller professionally drawn figures.

2. Using the attached table of tooth dimensions (same as in the associated textbook's appendices), mark off the overall peripheral tooth measurements for each of the gridded view boxes of the tooth. Note that the grid of the blank worksheet is larger than that shown with the professionally drawn tooth outlines to better enable the student to have room to work. Each square of grid equals 1 mm, so count off as many squares for each peripheral dimension (such as the mesiodistal diameter) as indicated from the table onto the proper area of the gridded worksheet.

3. To establish crown and root proportions, divide each gridded view box into two parts corresponding to these two dimensions, except for the incisal/occlusal view.

4. To indicate the height of contour, locate the approximate area of contact between the adjacent teeth and the area of greatest convexity on the labial/buccal, lingual/mesial, and distal surfaces as mentioned in the associated textbook.

5. To locate the root axis line (RAL), draw a line that exactly bisects the overall gridded box showing the overall crown and root measurements. The cementoenamel junction (CEJ) will then be bisected by the RAL. The root apex may or may not be located on this RAL, depending on the tooth's apex traits.

6. To locate the center of the cingulum or midpoint of the incisal edge, divide the crown and root (if included in that particular gridded view box) into imaginary thirds. Then place the root apex, cingulum, or incisal edge into proper perspective with respect to the other peripheral overall tooth dimensions such as the mesiodistal diameter.

7. To complete the crown outline, connect the heights of contour to the incisal/occlusal edge, to the CEJ, and to the other heights of contour. Any additional anatomical features such as mamelons, lobes, marginal ridges, depressions, and so forth, can be indicated upon completion of the crown outline.

8. To complete the root outline, follow the directions for developing the crown outline with the understanding that the cervical one third to one half of the root width generally approximates the cervical width of the crown before it starts to narrow considerably to form the root apex.

9. Shading or stippling of the features may now be added, if desired. An evaluation form for the drawings for use by both the student and instructor is also included in the workbook. Multiple copies of the form may be copied if needed.

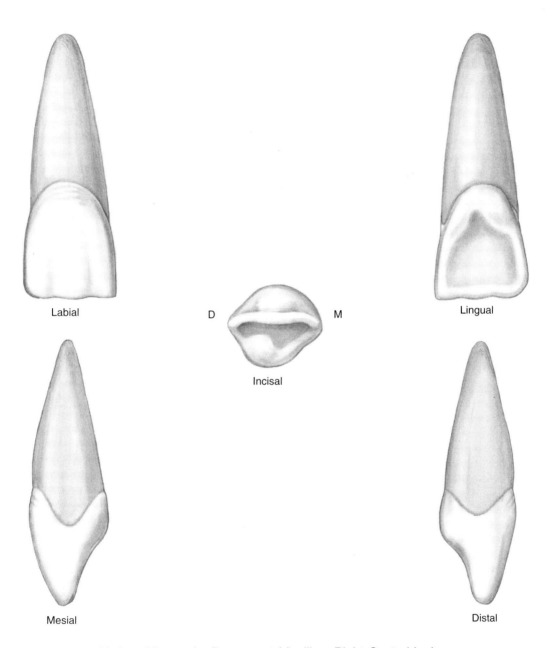

Labial

D   M

Incisal

Lingual

Mesial

Distal

Various Views of a Permanent Maxillary Right Central Incisor

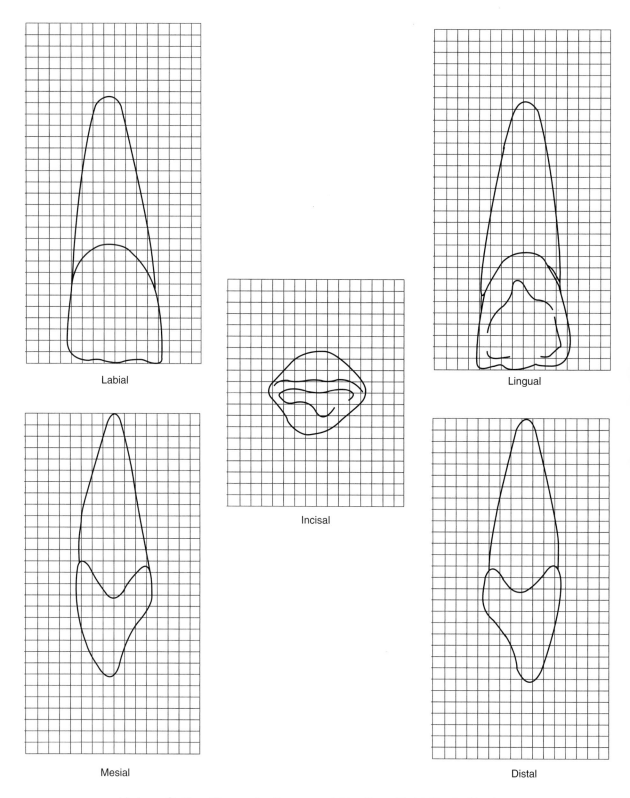

Labial

Lingual

Incisal

Mesial

Distal

Various Outline Views of a Permanent Maxillary Right Central Incisor

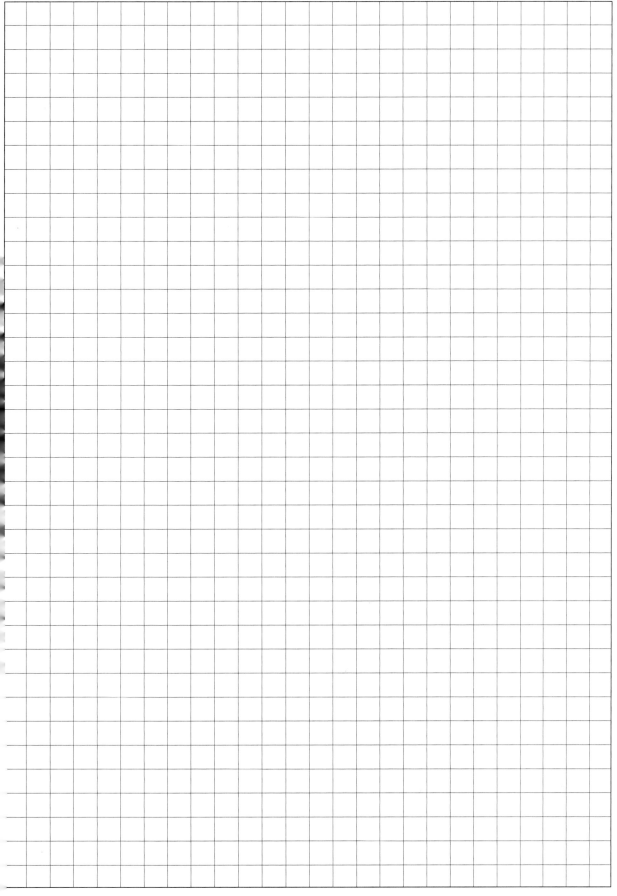

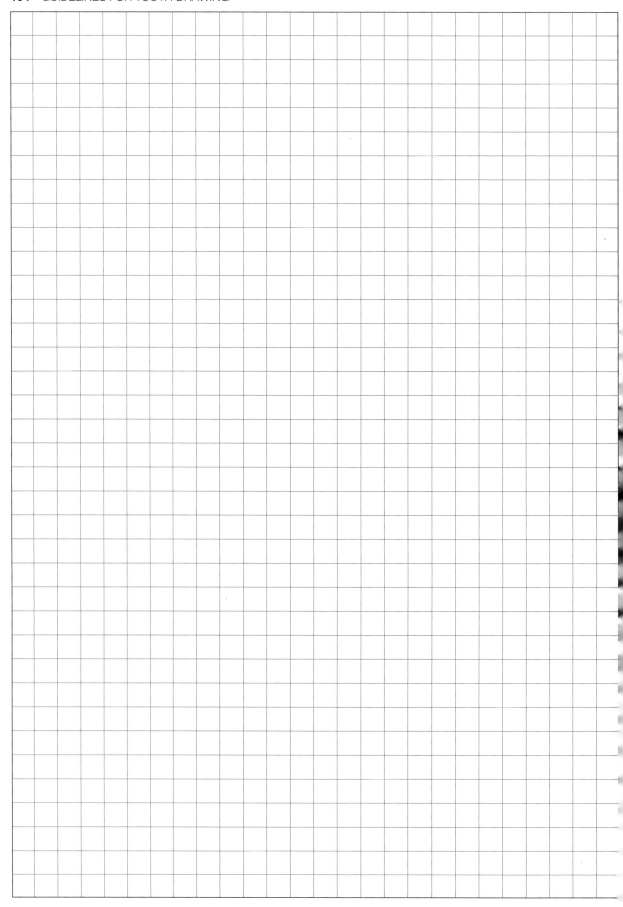

DIMENSIONS OF PERMANENT MAXILLARY CENTRAL INCISOR*

Cervico-incisal Length of Crown	10.5
Length of Root	13.0
Mesiodistal Diameter of Crown	8.5
Mesiodistal Diameter of CEJ	7.0
Labiolingual Diameter	7.0
Labiolingual Diameter of CEJ	6.0
Curvature of CEJ—Mesial	3.5
Curvature of CEJ—Distal	2.5

*In millimeters; adapted from Nelson SJ: *Wheeler's Dental Anatomy, Physiology, and Occlusions*, ed 9, WB Saunders, Philadelphia, 2009.

CEJ = cementoenamel junction

CHECKLIST FOR PERMANENT MAXILLARY CENTRAL INCISOR

Features Noted	Features Present
Crown Features	
Incisal edge, mamelons, distal offset cingulum, wide and shallow lingual fossa, longer mesial than distal marginal ridges, and linguoincisal edge	
Sharper MI incisal angle, rounder DI angle, and more pronounced mesial CEJ curvature	
Height of contour in cervical third	
Mesial contact is just cervical to the junction of occlusal and middle thirds	
Distal contact is at junction of incisal and middle thirds	
Root Features	
Single rooted, overall conical shape, rounded apex	
No proximal root concavities	

CEJ = cementoenamel junction; DI = distoincisal; MI = mesioincisal

Name _____   Tooth Number/Name _____

Date _____   Instructor Rating _____

DRAWING EVALUATION CHECKLIST

RATING SCALE

Fully Correct = 2 points   Major Error = 0 points
Minor Error = 1 point   Note: NA (non-appropriate)

SELF-EVALUATION RATING

Five Views	Clearly Drawn	Accurate Sizing	General Features Included	Specific Features Included
1. Facial View				
2. Lingual View				
3. Mesial View				
4. Distal View				
5. Incisal/ Occlusal View				

$$\text{Self-Evaluation Rating} = \frac{\text{Points received}}{\text{Points possible}} = \underline{\hspace{3cm}} = \underline{\hspace{2cm}} \%$$

INSTRUCTOR EVALUATION RATING

Five Views	Clearly Drawn	Accurate Sizing	General Features Included	Specific Features Included
1. Facial View				
2. Lingual View				
3. Mesial View				
4. Distal View				
5. Incisal/ Occlusal View				

$$\text{Instructor Evaluation Rating} = \frac{\text{Points received}}{\text{Points possible}} = \underline{\hspace{3cm}} = \underline{\hspace{2cm}} \%$$

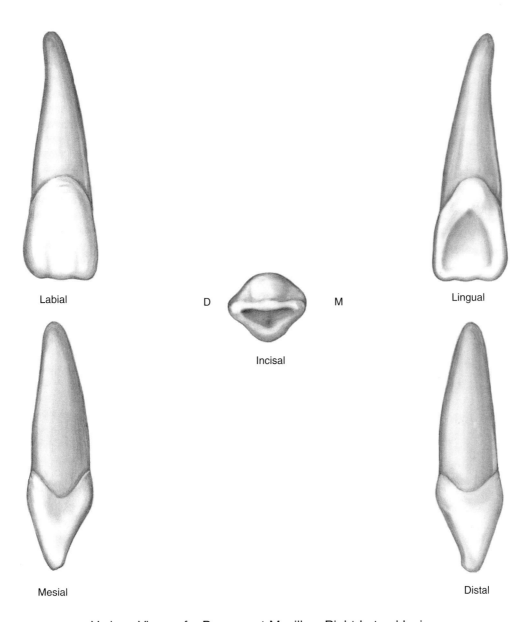

Labial

D M

Incisal

Lingual

Mesial

Distal

Various Views of a Permanent Maxillary Right Lateral Incisor

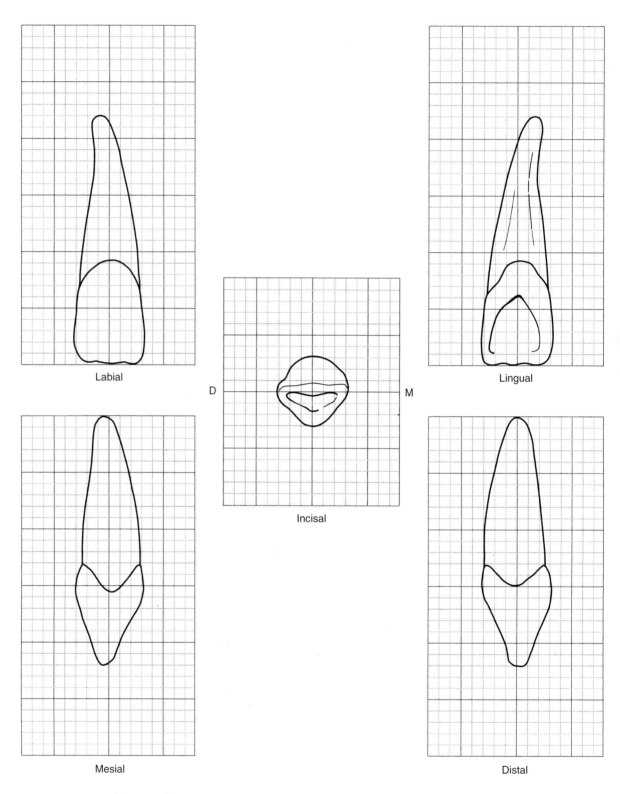

Labial

D   M

Incisal

Lingual

Mesial

Distal

Various Outline Views of a Permanent Maxillary Right Lateral Incisor

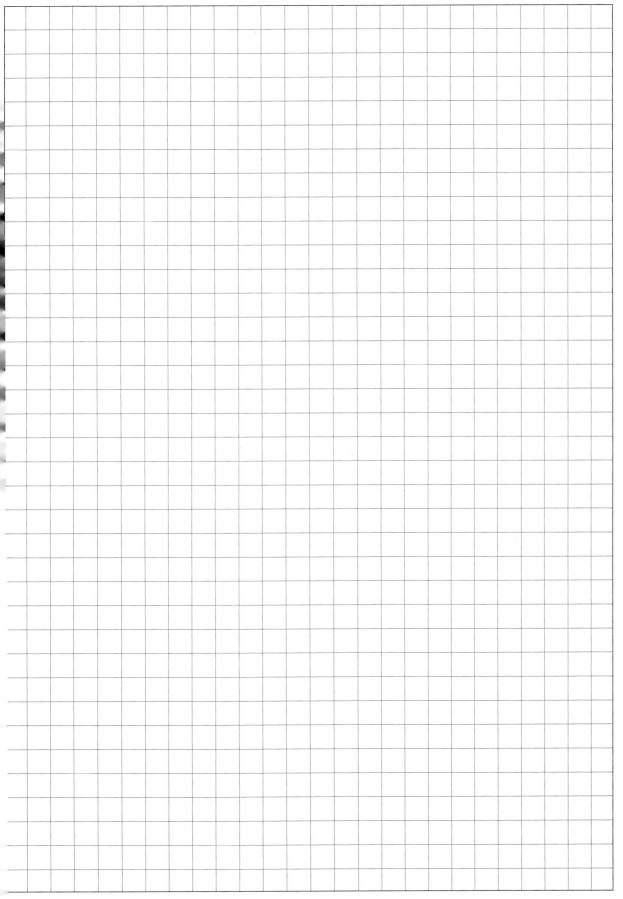

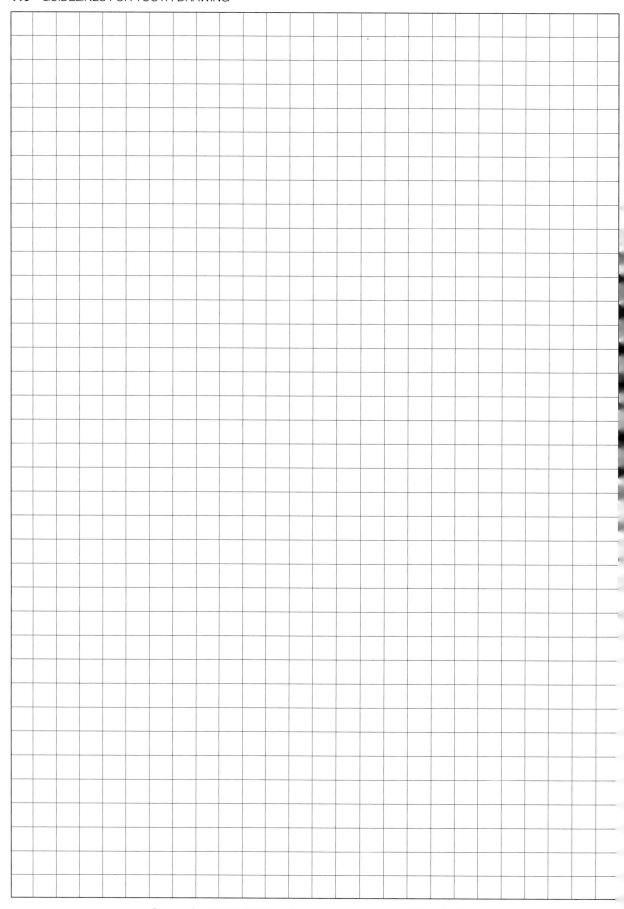

DIMENSIONS OF PERMANENT MAXILLARY LATERAL INCISOR*

Cervico-incisal Length of Crown	9.0
Length of Root	13.0
Mesiodistal Diameter of Crown	6.5
Mesiodistal Diameter of CEJ	5.0
Labiolingual Diameter	6.0
Labiolingual Diameter of CEJ	5.0
Curvature of CEJ—Mesial	3.0
Curvature of CEJ—Distal	2.0

*In millimeters; adapted from Nelson SJ: *Wheeler's Dental Anatomy, Physiology, and Occlusions*, ed 9, WB Saunders, Philadelphia, 2009.

CEJ = cementoenamel junction

CHECKLIST FOR PERMANENT MAXILLARY LATERAL INCISOR

Features Noted	Features Present
Crown Features	
Incisal edge, mamelons, centered and narrow cingulum, deep lingual fossa, pronounced marginal ridges, and linguoincisal ridge	
Sharper MI incisal angle, rounder DI angle, and more pronounced mesial CEJ curvature	
Height of contour in cervical third	
Mesial contact is just cervical to the junction of occlusal and middle thirds	
Distal contact is at middle third or junction with incisal third	
Root Features	
Single rooted, overall conical shape, root curve to the distal, with sharp apex	
No proximal root concavities and the same or longer than central, yet thinner	

CEJ = cementoenamel junction; DI = distoincisal; MI = mesioincisal

Name _____   Tooth Number/Name _____

Date _____   Instructor Rating _____

DRAWING EVALUATION CHECKLIST

RATING SCALE

Fully Correct = 2 points   Major Error = 0 points
Minor Error = 1 point   Note: NA (non-appropriate)

SELF-EVALUATION RATING

Five Views	Clearly Drawn	Accurate Sizing	General Features Included	Specific Features Included
1. Facial View				
2. Lingual View				
3. Mesial View				
4. Distal View				
5. Incisal/ Occlusal View				

$$\text{Self-Evaluation Rating} = \frac{\text{Points received}}{\text{Points possible}} = \underline{\hspace{2cm}} = \underline{\hspace{1.5cm}} \%$$

INSTRUCTOR EVALUATION RATING

Five Views	Clearly Drawn	Accurate Sizing	General Features Included	Specific Features Included
1. Facial View				
2. Lingual View				
3. Mesial View				
4. Distal View				
5. Incisal/ Occlusal View				

$$\text{Instructor Evaluation Rating} = \frac{\text{Points received}}{\text{Points possible}} = \underline{\hspace{2cm}} = \underline{\hspace{1.5cm}} \%$$

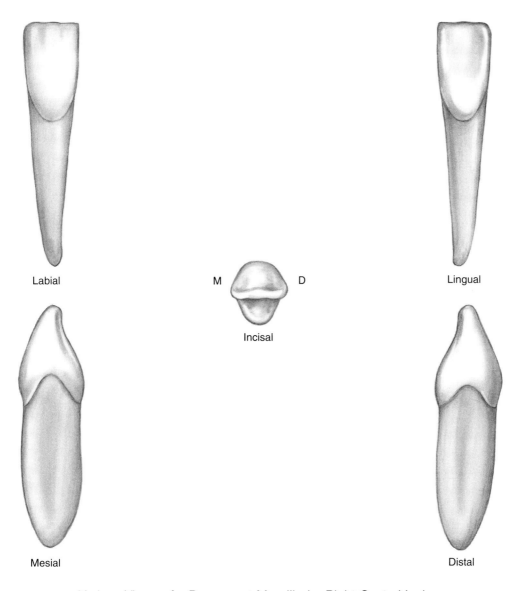

Labial

Lingual

M $\quad$ D

Incisal

Mesial

Distal

Various Views of a Permanent Mandibular Right Central Incisor

Labial

Lingual

Incisal

Mesial

Distal

Various Outline Views of a Permanent Mandibular Right Central Incisor

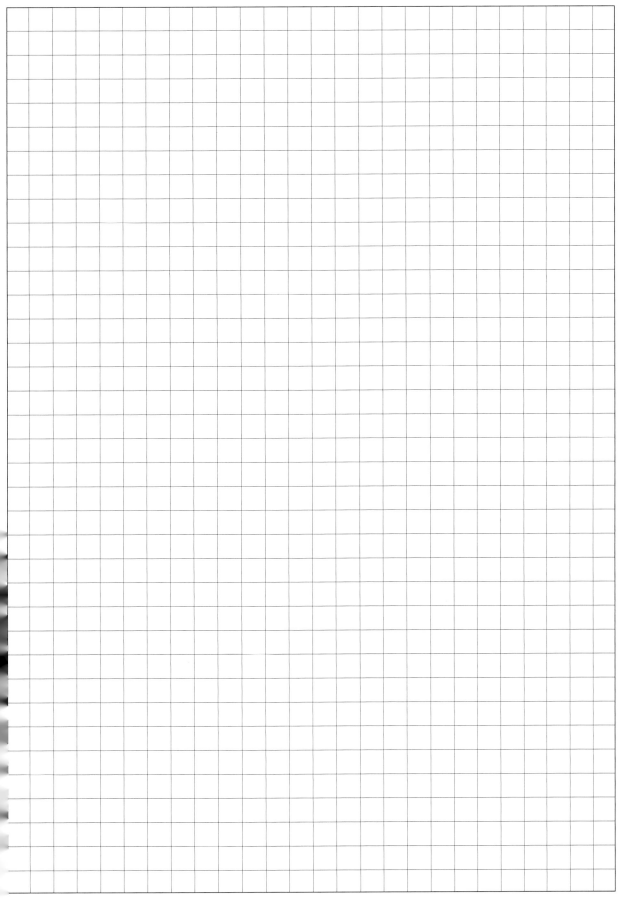

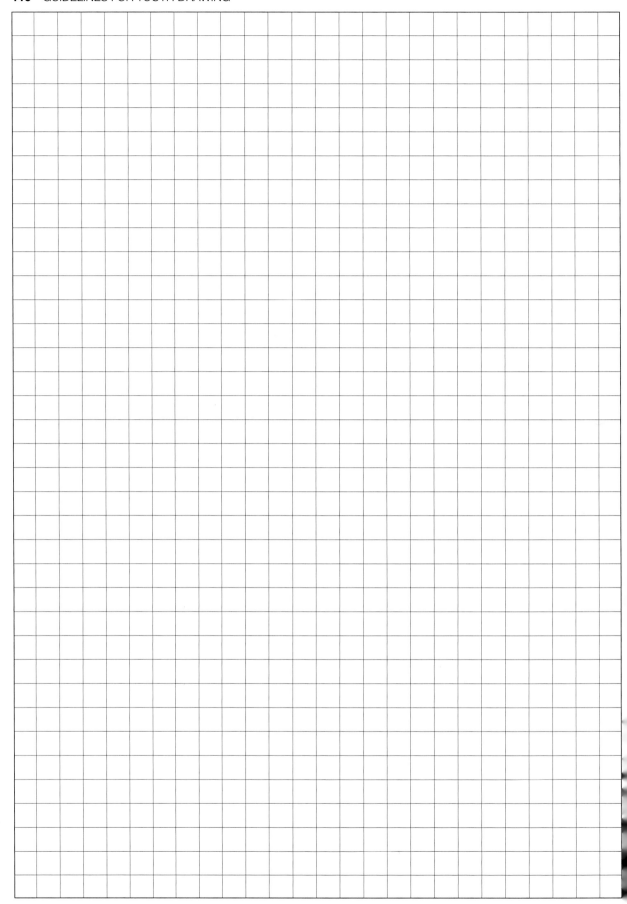

DIMENSIONS OF PERMANENT MANDIBULAR CENTRAL INCISOR*	
Cervico-incisal Length of Crown	Buccal: 9.0 Lingual: 9.5
Length of Root	12.5
Mesiodistal Diameter of Crown	5.0
Mesiodistal Diameter of CEJ	3.5
Labiolingual Diameter	6.0
Labiolingual Diameter of CEJ	5.3
Curvature of CEJ—Mesial	3.0
Curvature of CEJ—Distal	2.0

*In millimeters; adapted from Nelson SJ: *Wheeler's Dental Anatomy, Physiology, and Occlusions*, ed 9, WB Saunders, Philadelphia, 2009.

CEJ = cementoenamel junction

CHECKLIST FOR PERMANENT MANDIBULAR CENTRAL INCISOR	
Features Noted	**Features Present**
Crown Features	
Bilaterally symmetrical	
Incisal edge, mamelons, small centered cingulum, subtle lingual fossa, and equal subtle marginal ridges	
Sharper MI incisal angle, rounder DI angle, and more pronounced mesial CEJ curvature	
Height of contour in cervical third	
Mesial contact is just cervical to the junction of occlusal and middle thirds	
Distal contact is at incisal third	
Root Features	
Single rooted, with root longer than the crown	
Proximal root concavities give double-rooted appearance	

CEJ = cementoenamel junction; DI = distoincisal; MI = mesioincisal

Name _____   Tooth Number/Name _____

Date _____   Instructor Rating _____

DRAWING EVALUATION CHECKLIST

RATING SCALE

Fully Correct = 2 points   Major Error = 0 points
Minor Error = 1 point   Note: NA (non-appropriate)

SELF-EVALUATION RATING

Five Views	Clearly Drawn	Accurate Sizing	General Features Included	Specific Features Included
1. Facial View				
2. Lingual View				
3. Mesial View				
4. Distal View				
5. Incisal/ Occlusal View				

Self-Evaluation Rating = $\dfrac{\text{Points received}}{\text{Points possible}}$ = _____ = _____ %

INSTRUCTOR EVALUATION RATING

Five Views	Clearly Drawn	Accurate Sizing	General Features Included	Specific Features Included
1. Facial View				
2. Lingual View				
3. Mesial View				
4. Distal View				
5. Incisal/ Occlusal View				

Instructor Evaluation Rating = $\dfrac{\text{Points received}}{\text{Points possible}}$ = _____ = _____ %

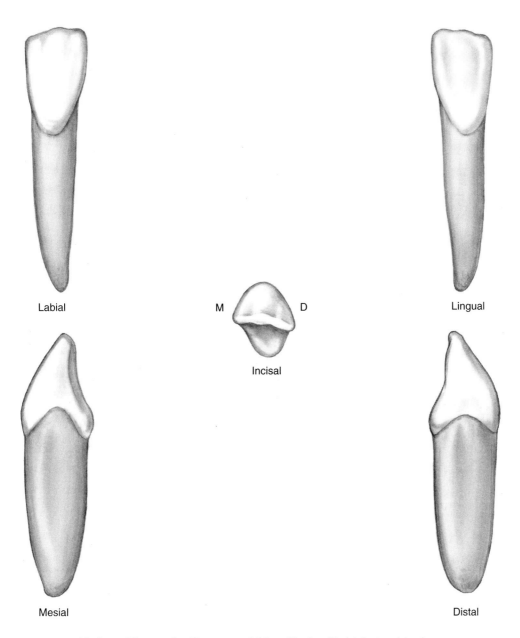

Labial

M   D

Incisal

Lingual

Mesial

Distal

Various Views of a Permanent Mandibular Right Lateral Incisor

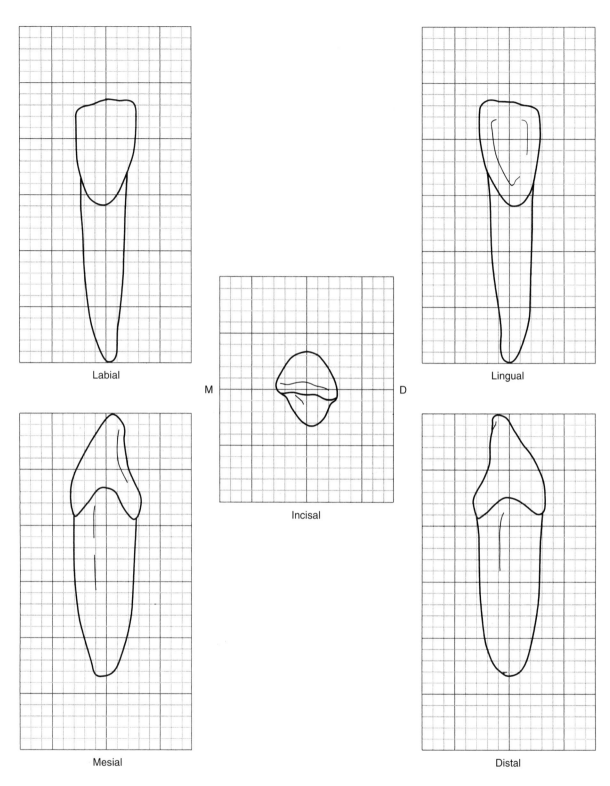

Labial

Lingual

M   D

Incisal

Mesial

Distal

Various Outline Views of a Permanent Mandibular Right Lateral Incisor

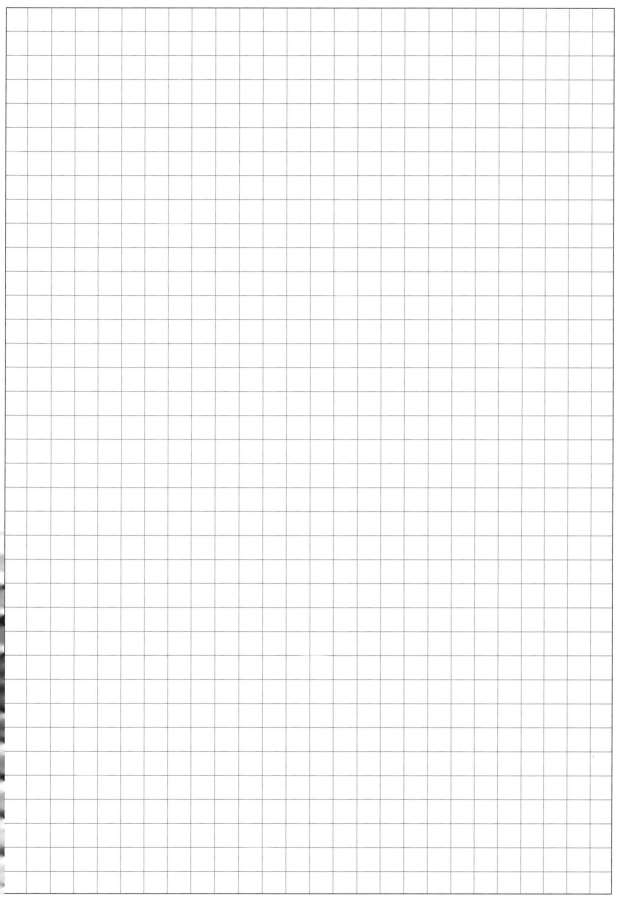

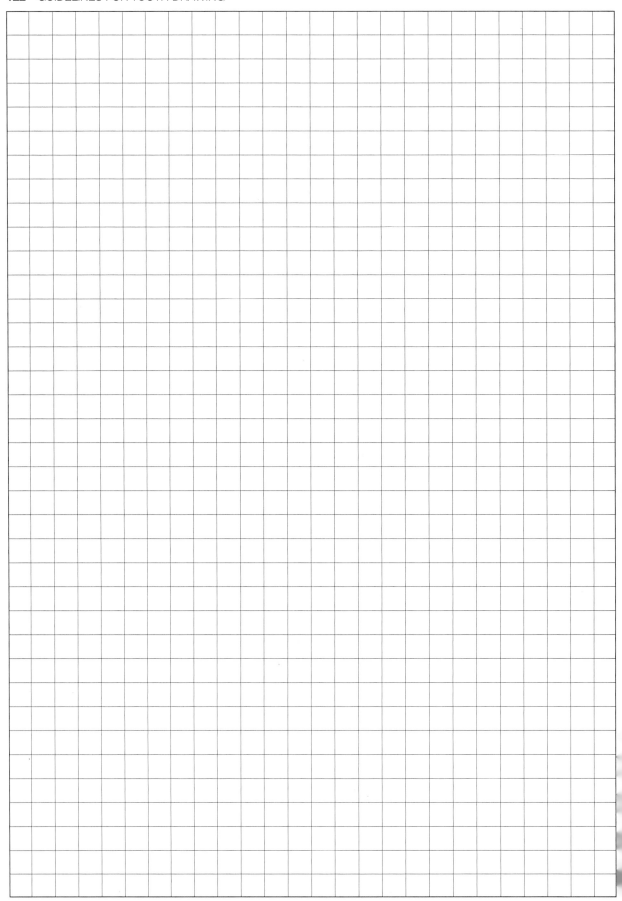

DIMENSIONS OF PERMANENT MANDIBULAR LATERAL INCISOR*

Cervico-incisal Length of Crown	Buccal: 9.5 Lingual: 10.0
Length of Root	14.0
Mesiodistal Diameter of Crown	5.5
Mesiodistal Diameter of CEJ	4.0
Labiolingual Diameter	6.5
Labiolingual Diameter of CEJ	5.8
Curvature of CEJ—Mesial	3.0
Curvature of CEJ—Distal	2.0

*In millimeters; adapted from Nelson SJ: *Wheeler's Dental Anatomy, Physiology, and Occlusions*, ed 9, WB Saunders, Philadelphia, 2009.

CEJ = cementoenamel junction

CHECKLIST FOR PERMANENT MANDIBULAR LATERAL INCISOR

Features Noted	Features Present
Crown Features	
Larger than central and not bilaterally symmetrical, and appears twisted distally	
Incisal edge, mamelons, small distally displaced cingulum, lingual fossa, and moderate mesial marginal ridge longer than distal	
Sharper MI incisal angle, rounder DI angle, and more pronounced mesial CEJ curvature	
Height of contour in cervical third	
Mesial contact is just cervical to the junction of occlusal and middle thirds	
Distal contact is at incisal third	
Root Features	
Single rooted, with root longer than the crown	
Proximal root concavities give double-rooted appearance	

CEJ = cementoenamel junction; DI = distoincisal; MI = mesioincisal

Name _____ Tooth Number/Name _____

Date _____ Instructor Rating _____

DRAWING EVALUATION CHECKLIST

RATING SCALE
Fully Correct = 2 points   Major Error = 0 points
Minor Error = 1 point   Note: NA (non-appropriate)

SELF-EVALUATION RATING

Five Views	Clearly Drawn	Accurate Sizing	General Features Included	Specific Features Included
1. Facial View				
2. Lingual View				
3. Mesial View				
4. Distal View				
5. Incisal/ Occlusal View				

Self-Evaluation Rating = $\frac{\text{Points received}}{\text{Points possible}}$ = _____ = _____ %

INSTRUCTOR EVALUATION RATING

Five Views	Clearly Drawn	Accurate Sizing	General Features Included	Specific Features Included
1. Facial View				
2. Lingual View				
3. Mesial View				
4. Distal View				
5. Incisal/ Occlusal View				

Instructor Evaluation Rating = $\frac{\text{Points received}}{\text{Points possible}}$ = _____ = _____ %

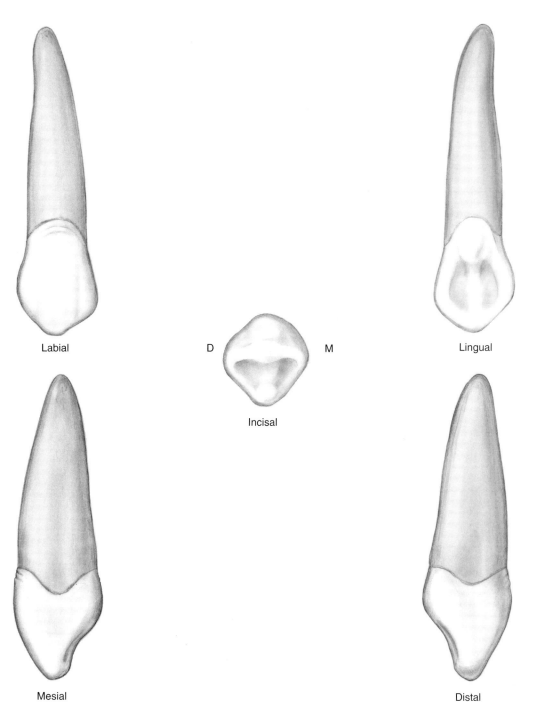

Labial

D · M

Incisal

Lingual

Mesial

Distal

Various Views of a Permanent Maxillary Right Canine

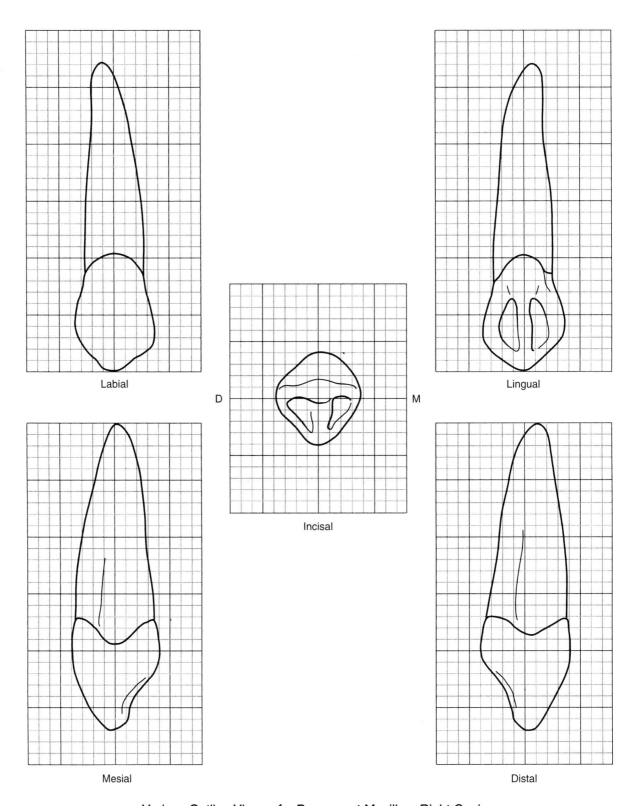

Labial

Lingual

D   M

Incisal

Mesial

Distal

Various Outline Views of a Permanent Maxillary Right Canine

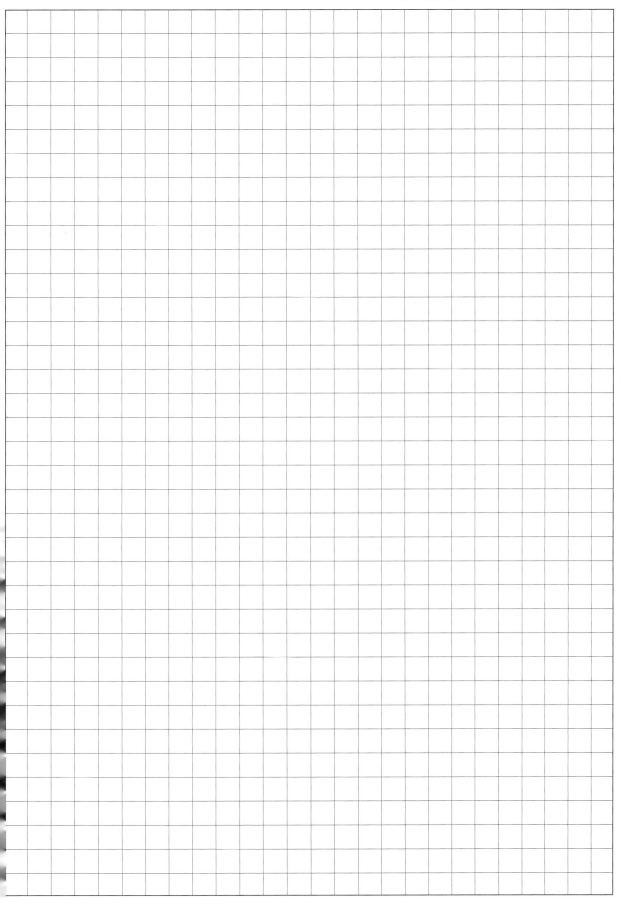

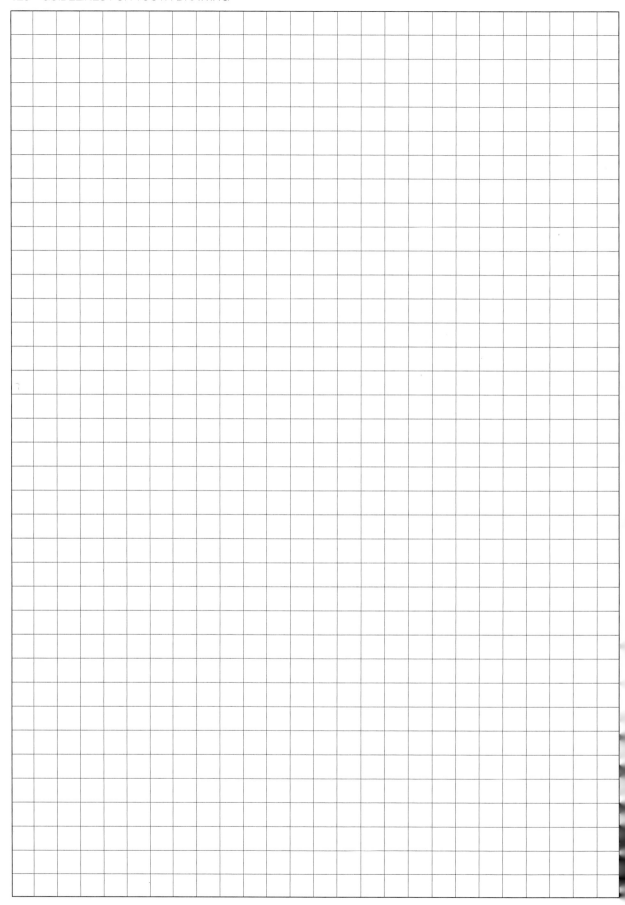

DIMENSIONS OF PERMANENT MAXILLARY CANINE*

Cervico-incisal Length of Crown	10.0
Length of Root	17.0
Mesiodistal Diameter of Crown	7.5
Mesiodistal Diameter of CEJ	5.5
Labiolingual Diameter	8.0
Labiolingual Diameter of CEJ	7.0
Curvature of CEJ—Mesial	2.5
Curvature of CEJ—Distal	1.5

*In millimeters; adapted from Nelson SJ: *Wheeler's Dental Anatomy, Physiology, and Occlusions*, ed 9, WB Saunders, Philadelphia, 2009.

CEJ = cementoenamel junction

CHECKLIST FOR PERMANENT MAXILLARY CANINE

Features Noted	Features Present
Crown Features	
Single cusp, with sharp cusp tip and slopes, labial ridge	
Shorter mesial cusp slope, more cervical contact on distal, more pronounced mesial CEJ curvature	
Shorter distal outline on labial view with depression between the distal contact and CEJ	
Prominent lingual anatomy with marginal ridges and lingual ridge, cingulum, and lingual fossae	
Height of contour for buccal is cervical third and for lingual is middle third	
Mesial contact is at junction of incisal third and middle thirds	
Distal contact is at middle third	
Root Features	
Long, thick single root with proximal root concavities	
Blunt root apex	

CEJ = cementoenamel junction

Name _____   Tooth Number/Name _____

Date _____   Instructor Rating _____

DRAWING EVALUATION CHECKLIST

RATING SCALE

Fully Correct = 2 points   Major Error = 0 points
Minor Error = 1 point   Note: NA (non-appropriate)

SELF-EVALUATION RATING

Five Views	Clearly Drawn	Accurate Sizing	General Features Included	Specific Features Included
1. Facial View				
2. Lingual View				
3. Mesial View				
4. Distal View				
5. Incisal/ Occlusal View				

$$\text{Self-Evaluation Rating} = \frac{\text{Points received}}{\text{Points possible}} = \underline{\hspace{3cm}} = \underline{\hspace{2cm}} \%$$

INSTRUCTOR EVALUATION RATING

Five Views	Clearly Drawn	Accurate Sizing	General Features Included	Specific Features Included
1. Facial View				
2. Lingual View				
3. Mesial View				
4. Distal View				
5. Incisal/ Occlusal View				

$$\text{Instructor Evaluation Rating} = \frac{\text{Points received}}{\text{Points possible}} = \underline{\hspace{3cm}} = \underline{\hspace{2cm}} \%$$

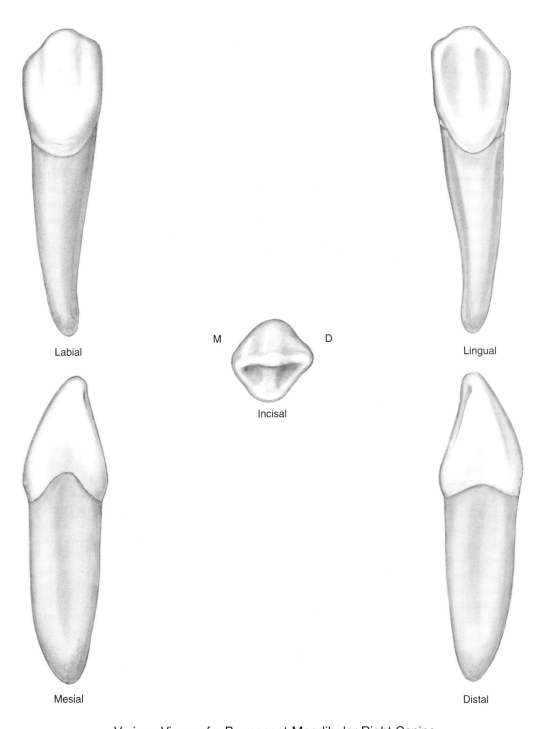

Labial

Lingual

M   D

Incisal

Mesial

Distal

Various Views of a Permanent Mandibular Right Canine

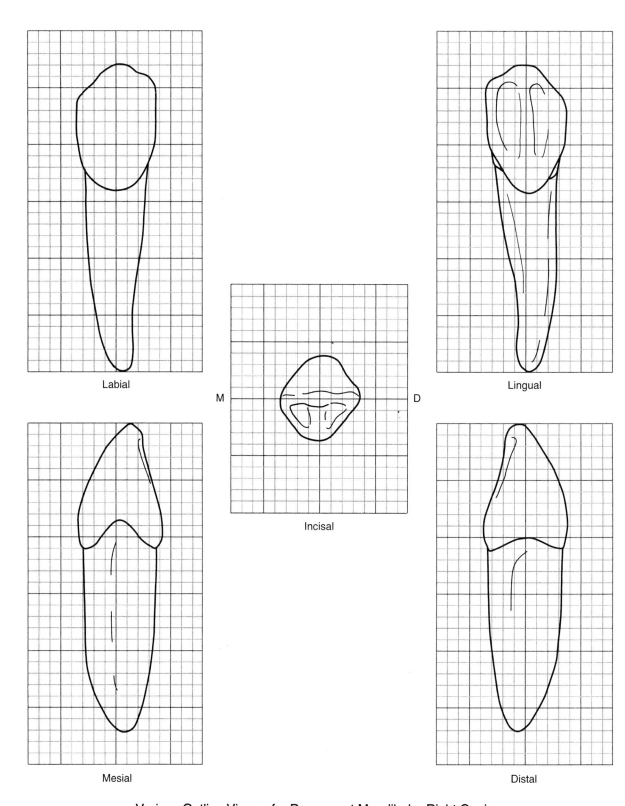

Labial

Lingual

M   D

Incisal

Mesial

Distal

Various Outline Views of a Permanent Mandibular Right Canine

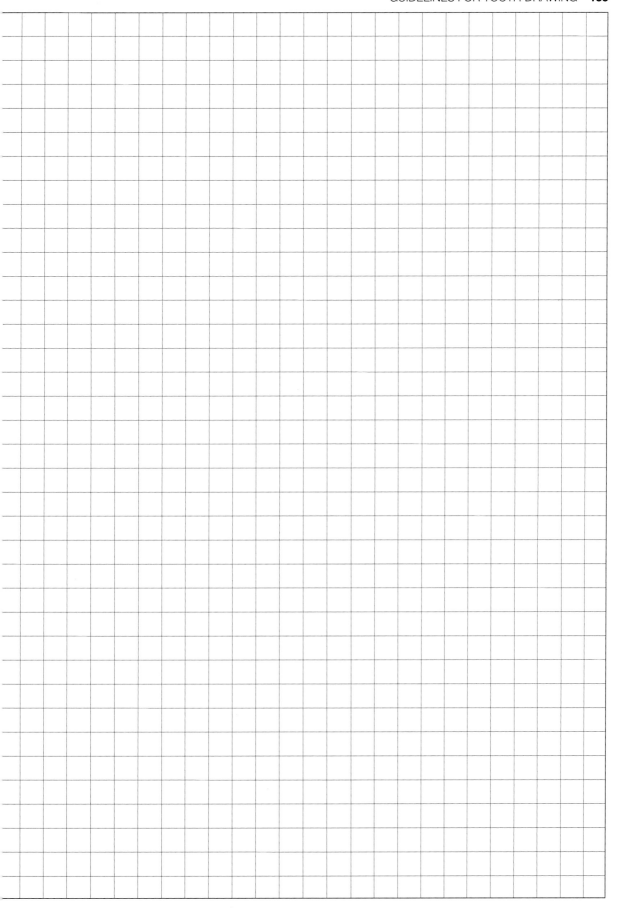

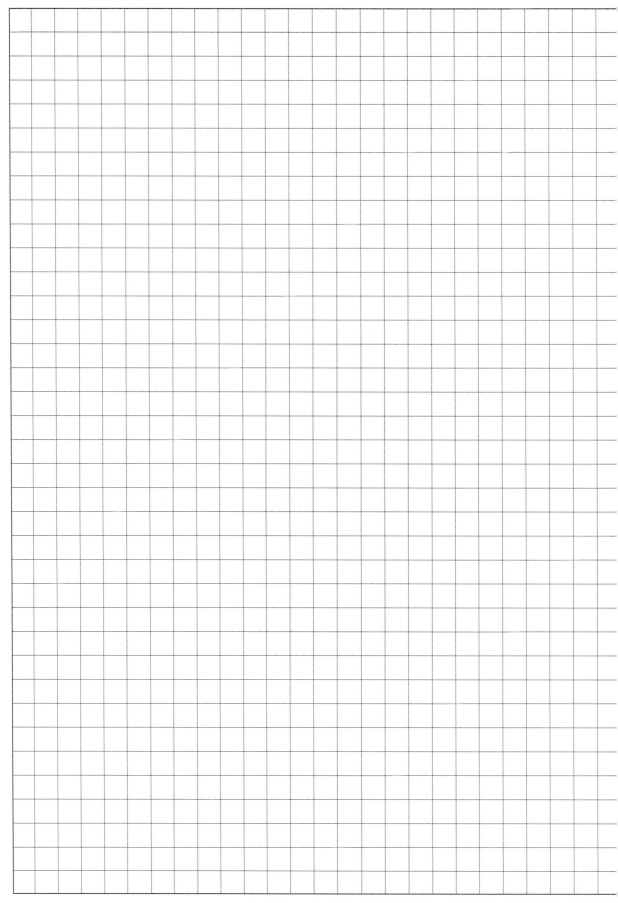

DIMENSIONS OF PERMANENT MANDIBULAR CANINE*

Cervico-incisal Length of Crown	11.0
Length of Root	16.0
Mesiodistal Diameter of Crown	7.0
Mesiodistal Diameter of CEJ	5.5
Labiolingual Diameter	7.5
Labiolingual Diameter of CEJ	7.0
Curvature of CEJ—Mesial	2.5
Curvature of CEJ—Distal	1.0

*In millimeters; adapted from Nelson SJ: *Wheeler's Dental Anatomy, Physiology, and Occlusions,* ed 9, WB Saunders, Philadelphia, 2009.

CEJ = cementoenamel junction

CHECKLIST FOR PERMANENT MANDIBULAR CANINE

Features Noted	Features Present
Crown Features	
Single cusp, with less sharp cusp tip and slopes, labial ridge	
Shorter mesial cusp slope, more cervical contact on distal, more pronounced mesial CEJ curvature	
Shorter and rounder distal outline on labial view, with a shorter mesial slope than distal	
Smoother lingual anatomy	
Height of contour for buccal is cervical third and for lingual is middle third	
Mesial contact is at incisal thirds	
Distal contact is at junction of incisal and middle thirds	
Root Features	
Long, thick single root with proximal root concavities and with pointed apex	
Developmental depressions on mesial and distal give tooth double-rooted appearance	

CEJ = cementoenamel junction

Name _____   Tooth Number/Name _____

Date _____   Instructor Rating _____

DRAWING EVALUATION CHECKLIST

RATING SCALE
Fully Correct = 2 points   Major Error = 0 points
Minor Error = 1 point   Note: NA (non-appropriate)

SELF-EVALUATION RATING

Five Views	Clearly Drawn	Accurate Sizing	General Features Included	Specific Features Included
1. Facial View				
2. Lingual View				
3. Mesial View				
4. Distal View				
5. Incisal/ Occlusal View				

Self-Evaluation Rating = $\frac{\text{Points received}}{\text{Points possible}}$ = _____ = _____ %

INSTRUCTOR EVALUATION RATING

Five Views	Clearly Drawn	Accurate Sizing	General Features Included	Specific Features Included
1. Facial View				
2. Lingual View				
3. Mesial View				
4. Distal View				
5. Incisal/ Occlusal View				

Instructor Evaluation Rating = $\frac{\text{Points received}}{\text{Points possible}}$ = _____ = _____ %

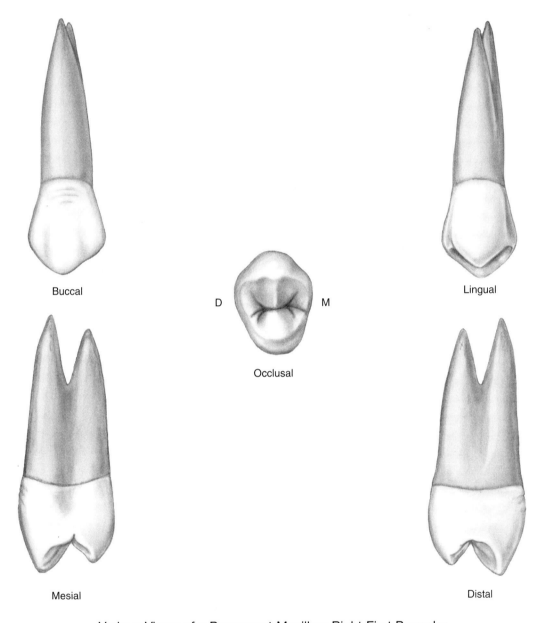

Buccal

Lingual

D M

Occlusal

Mesial

Distal

Various Views of a Permanent Maxillary Right First Premolar

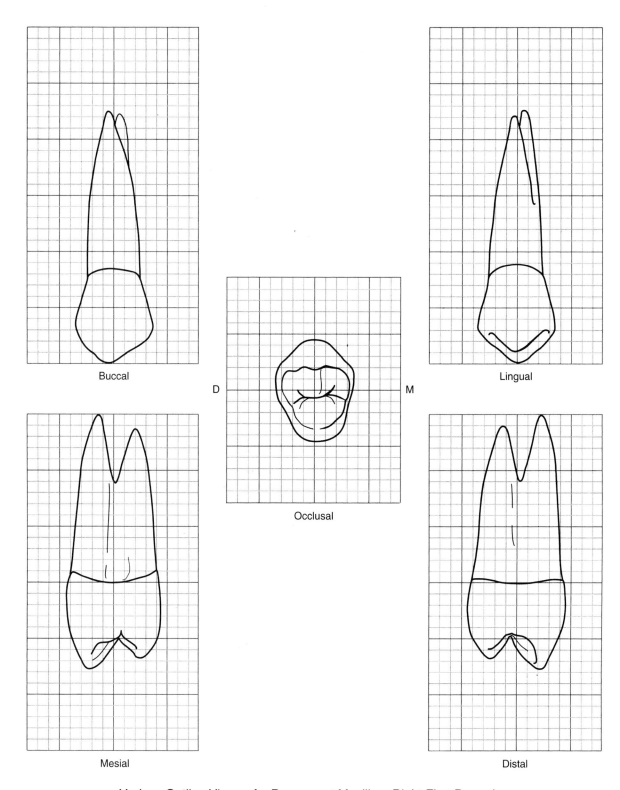

Buccal

Lingual

D

M

Occlusal

Mesial

Distal

Various Outline Views of a Permanent Maxillary Right First Premolar

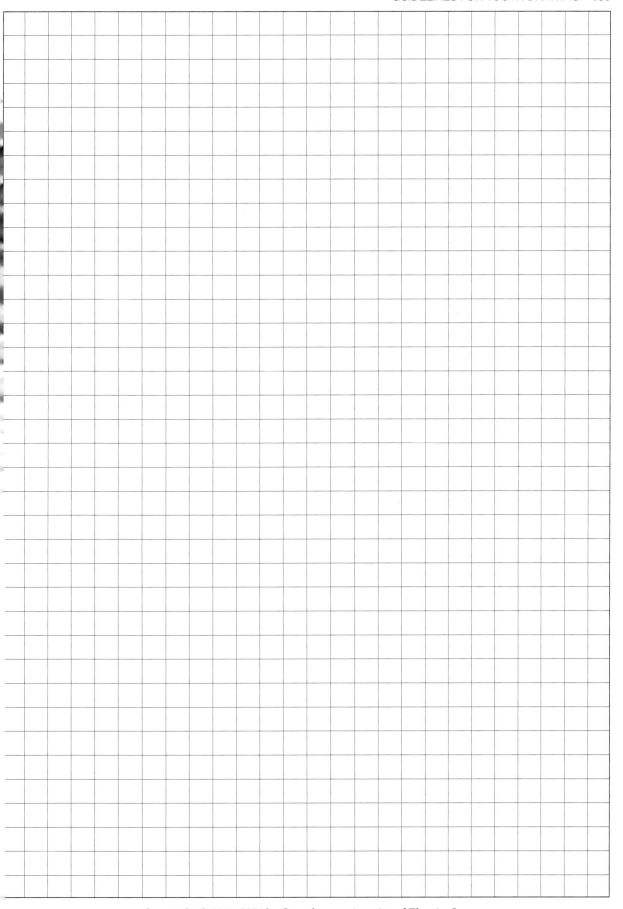

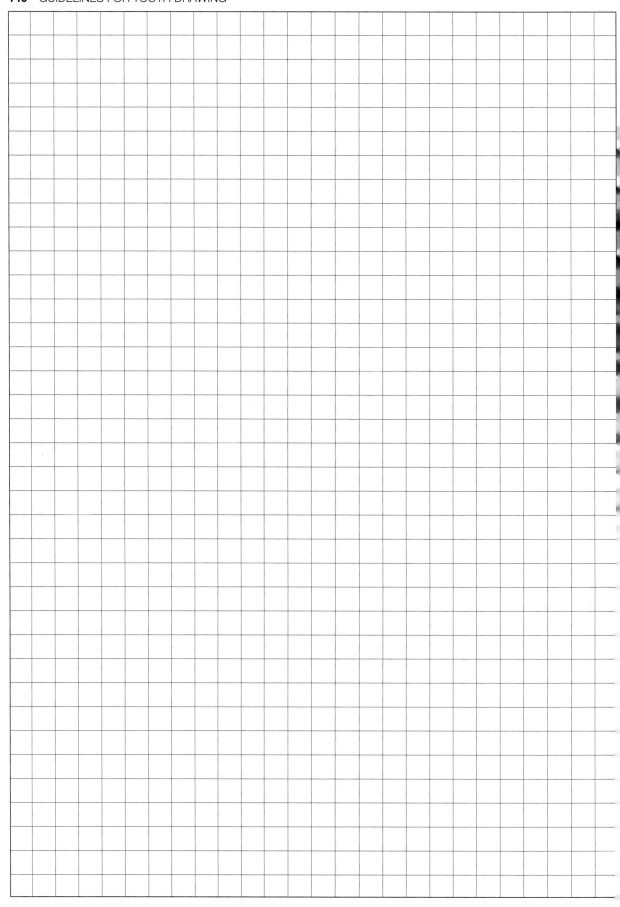

DIMENSIONS OF PERMANENT MAXILLARY FIRST PREMOLAR*

Cervico-incisal Length of Crown	8.5
Length of Root	14.0
Mesiodistal Diameter of Crown	7.0
Mesiodistal Diameter of CEJ	5.0
Buccolingual Diameter	9.0
Buccolingual Diameter of CEJ	8.0
Curvature of CEJ—Mesial	1.0
Curvature of CEJ—Distal	0.0

*In millimeters; adapted from Nelson SJ: *Wheeler's Dental Anatomy, Physiology, and Occlusions*, ed 9, WB Saunders, Philadelphia, 2009.

CEJ = cementoenamel junction

CHECKLIST FOR PERMANENT MAXILLARY FIRST PREMOLAR

Features Noted	Features Present
Crown Features	
Buccal cusp longer of two with buccal ridge	
Occlusal table with marginal ridges and cusps, with tips, ridges, inclined planes, and grooves (long central groove), fossae, pits	
Longer mesial cusp slope, mesial marginal groove, mesial developmental depression, deeper mesial CEJ curvature	
Mesial and distal contact is just cervical to the junction of occlusal and middle thirds	
Root Features	
Bifurcated with root trunk	
Proximal root concavities	

CEJ = cementoenamel junction

Name _____   Tooth Number/Name _____

Date _____   Instructor Rating _____

DRAWING EVALUATION CHECKLIST

RATING SCALE

Fully Correct = 2 points   Major Error = 0 points
Minor Error = 1 point   Note: NA (non-appropriate)

SELF-EVALUATION RATING

Five Views	Clearly Drawn	Accurate Sizing	General Features Included	Specific Features Included
1. Facial View				
2. Lingual View				
3. Mesial View				
4. Distal View				
5. Incisal/ Occlusal View				

Self-Evaluation Rating $= \dfrac{\text{Points received}}{\text{Points possible}} =$ _____ $=$ _____ %

INSTRUCTOR EVALUATION RATING

Five Views	Clearly Drawn	Accurate Sizing	General Features Included	Specific Features Included
1. Facial View				
2. Lingual View				
3. Mesial View				
4. Distal View				
5. Incisal/ Occlusal View				

Instructor Evaluation Rating $= \dfrac{\text{Points received}}{\text{Points possible}} =$ _____ $=$ _____ %

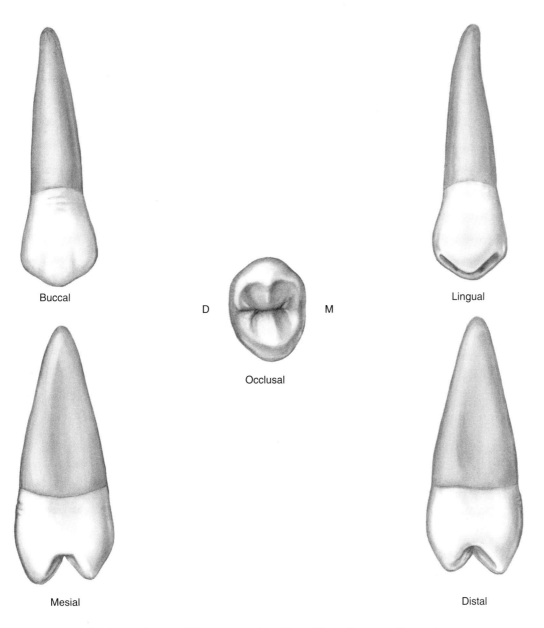

Buccal

Lingual

D   M

Occlusal

Mesial

Distal

Various Views of Permanent Maxillary Right Second Premolar

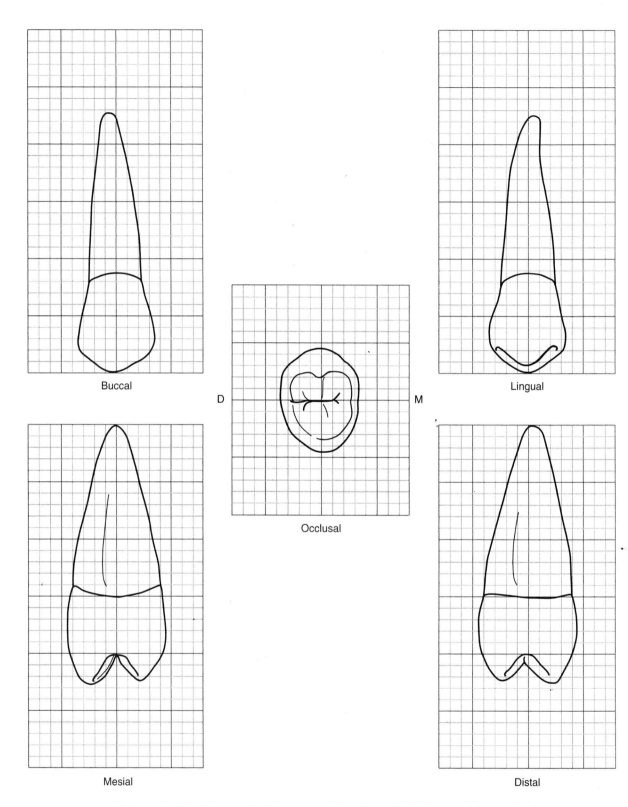

Buccal

Lingual

D   M

Occlusal

Mesial

Distal

Various Outline Views of a Permanent Maxillary Right Second Premolar

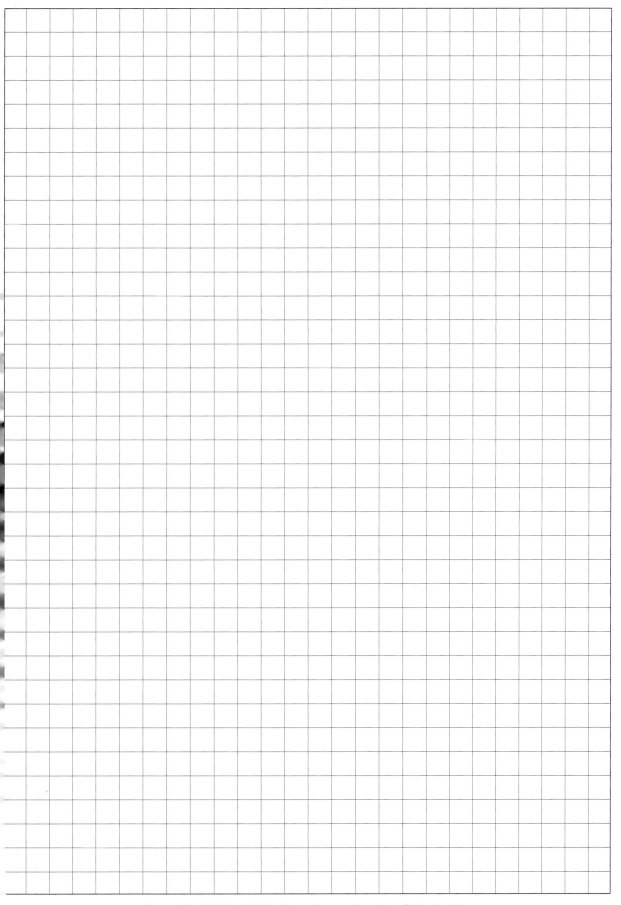

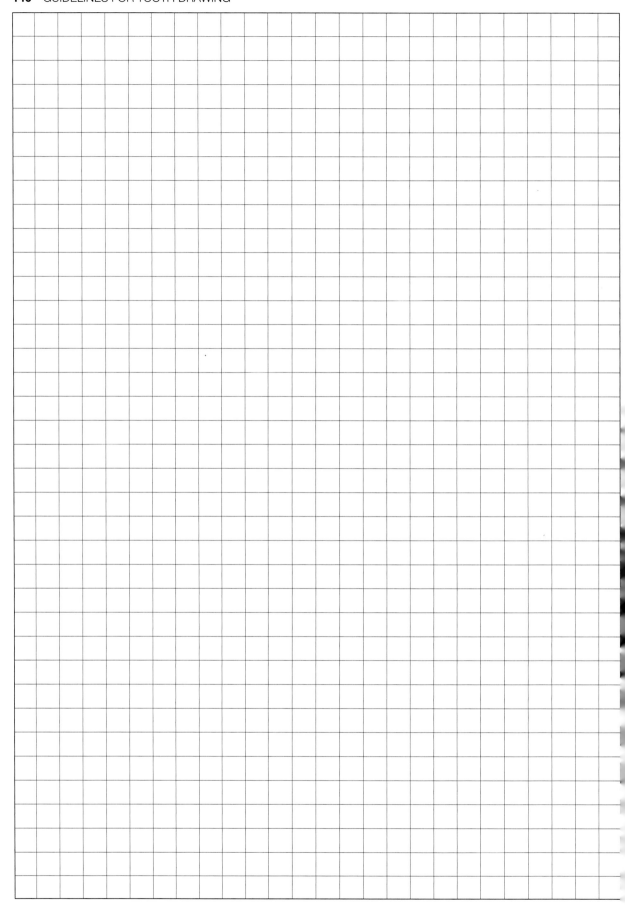

DIMENSIONS OF PERMANENT MAXILLARY SECOND PREMOLAR*	
Cervico-incisal Length of Crown	8.5
Length of Root	14.0
Mesiodistal Diameter of Crown	7.0
Mesiodistal Diameter of CEJ	5.0
Buccolingual Diameter	9.0
Buccolingual Diameter of CEJ	8.0
Curvature of CEJ—Mesial	1.0
Curvature of CEJ—Distal	0.0

*In millimeters; adapted from Nelson SJ: *Wheeler's Dental Anatomy, Physiology, and Occlusions,* ed 9, WB Saunders, Philadelphia, 2009.

CEJ = cementoenamel junction

CHECKLIST FOR PERMANENT MAXILLARY SECOND PREMOLAR	
Features Noted	**Features Present**
Crown Features	
Two cusps same length with buccal ridge	
Occlusal table with marginal ridges and cusps, with tips, ridges, inclined planes, and grooves (short central groove and increased supplemental grooves), fossae, pits	
Lingual cusp offset to the mesial	
Mesial and distal contact is just cervical to the junction of occlusal and middle thirds	
Root Features	
Single rooted	
Proximal root concavities	

CEJ = cementoenamel junction

Name _____   Tooth Number/Name _____

Date _____   Instructor Rating _____

DRAWING EVALUATION CHECKLIST

RATING SCALE
Fully Correct = 2 points   Major Error = 0 points
Minor Error = 1 point   Note: NA (non-appropriate)

SELF-EVALUATION RATING

Five Views	Clearly Drawn	Accurate Sizing	General Features Included	Specific Features Included
1. Facial View				
2. Lingual View				
3. Mesial View				
4. Distal View				
5. Incisal/ Occlusal View				

$$\text{Self-Evaluation Rating} = \frac{\text{Points received}}{\text{Points possible}} = \underline{\hspace{3cm}} = \underline{\hspace{2cm}} \%$$

INSTRUCTOR EVALUATION RATING

Five Views	Clearly Drawn	Accurate Sizing	General Features Included	Specific Features Included
1. Facial View				
2. Lingual View				
3. Mesial View				
4. Distal View				
5. Incisal/ Occlusal View				

$$\text{Instructor Evaluation Rating} = \frac{\text{Points received}}{\text{Points possible}} = \underline{\hspace{3cm}} = \underline{\hspace{2cm}} \%$$

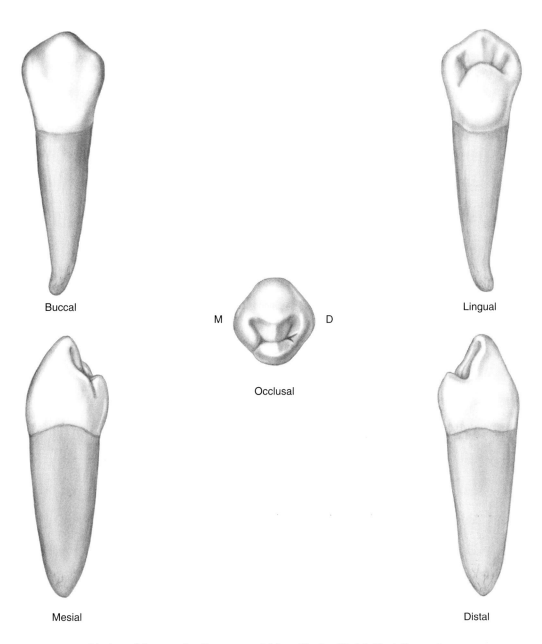

Buccal

Lingual

M   D

Occlusal

Mesial

Distal

Various Views of a Permanent Mandibular Right First Premolar

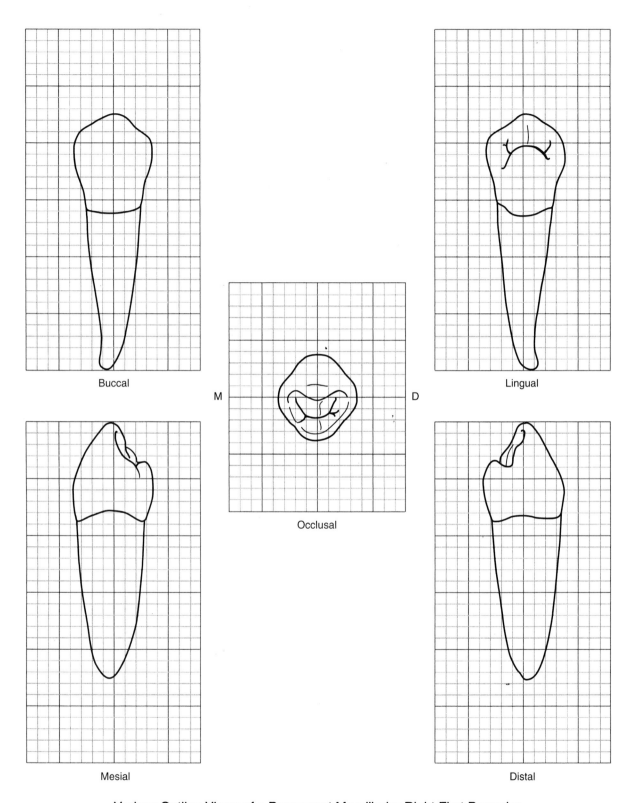

Buccal

Lingual

M

D

Occlusal

Mesial

Distal

Various Outline Views of a Permanent Mandibular Right First Premolar

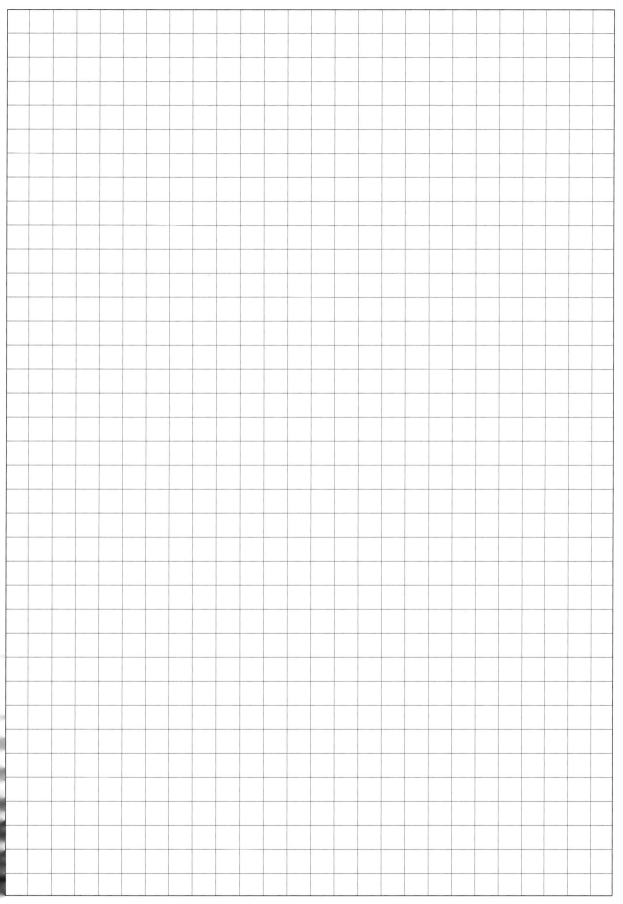

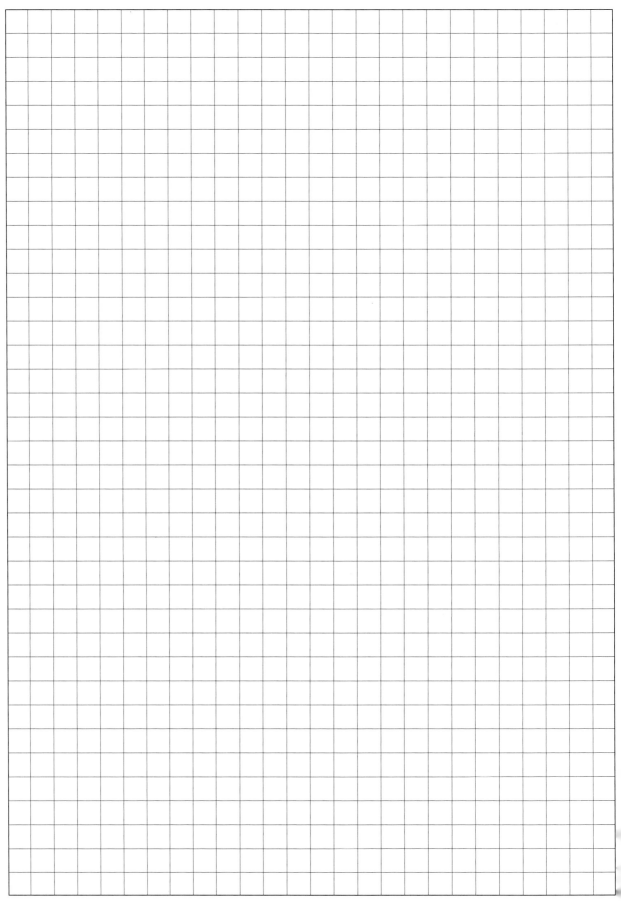

DIMENSIONS OF PERMANENT MANDIBULAR FIRST PREMOLAR*

Cervico-incisal Length of Crown	8.5
Length of Root	14.0
Mesiodistal Diameter of Crown	7.0
Mesiodistal Diameter of CEJ	5.0
Buccolingual Diameter	7.5
Buccolingual Diameter of CEJ	6.5
Curvature of CEJ—Mesial	1.0
Curvature of CEJ—Distal	0.0

*In millimeters; adapted from Nelson SJ: *Wheeler's Dental Anatomy, Physiology, and Occlusions,* ed 9, WB Saunders, Philadelphia, 2009.

CEJ = cementoenamel junction

CHECKLIST FOR PERMANENT MANDIBULAR FIRST PREMOLAR

Features Noted	Features Present
Crown Features	
Smaller lingual cusp of two with buccal ridge	
Occlusal table with marginal ridges and cusps, with tips, ridges, inclined planes, and grooves, fossae, pits	
Shorter mesial cusp slope, mesiolingual groove, deeper mesial CEJ curvature	
Mesial and distal contact is just cervical to the junction of occlusal and middle thirds	
Root Features	
Single rooted	
Proximal root concavities	

CEJ = cementoenamel junction

Name _____   Tooth Number/Name _____

Date _____   Instructor Rating _____

DRAWING EVALUATION CHECKLIST

RATING SCALE
Fully Correct = 2 points   Major Error = 0 points
Minor Error = 1 point   Note: NA (non-appropriate)

SELF-EVALUATION RATING

Five Views	Clearly Drawn	Accurate Sizing	General Features Included	Specific Features Included
1. Facial View				
2. Lingual View				
3. Mesial View				
4. Distal View				
5. Incisal/ Occlusal View				

Self-Evaluation Rating = $\frac{\text{Points received}}{\text{Points possible}}$ = _____ = _____ %

INSTRUCTOR EVALUATION RATING

Five Views	Clearly Drawn	Accurate Sizing	General Features Included	Specific Features Included
1. Facial View				
2. Lingual View				
3. Mesial View				
4. Distal View				
5. Incisal/ Occlusal View				

Instructor Evaluation Rating = $\frac{\text{Points received}}{\text{Points possible}}$ = _____ = _____ %

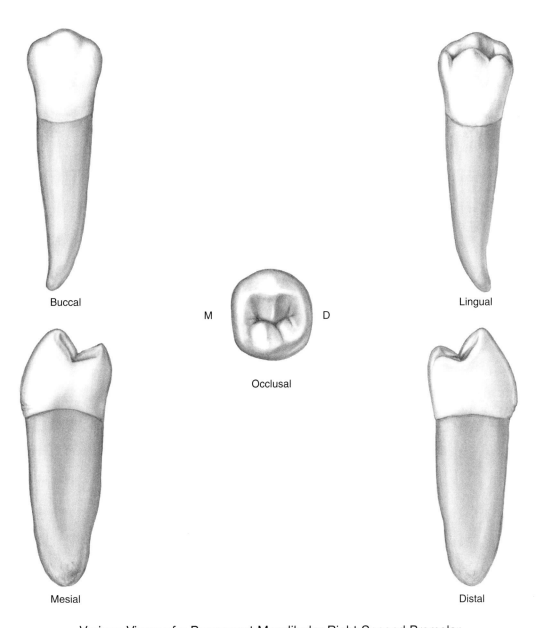

Buccal

M   D

Occlusal

Lingual

Mesial

Distal

Various Views of a Permanent Mandibular Right Second Premolar

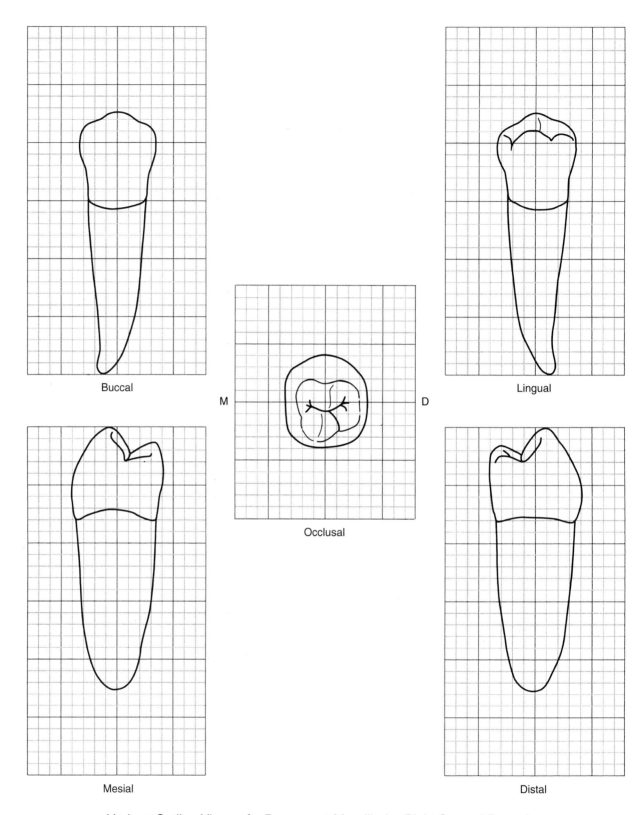

Buccal

Lingual

M

D

Occlusal

Mesial

Distal

Various Outline Views of a Permanent Mandibular Right Second Premolar

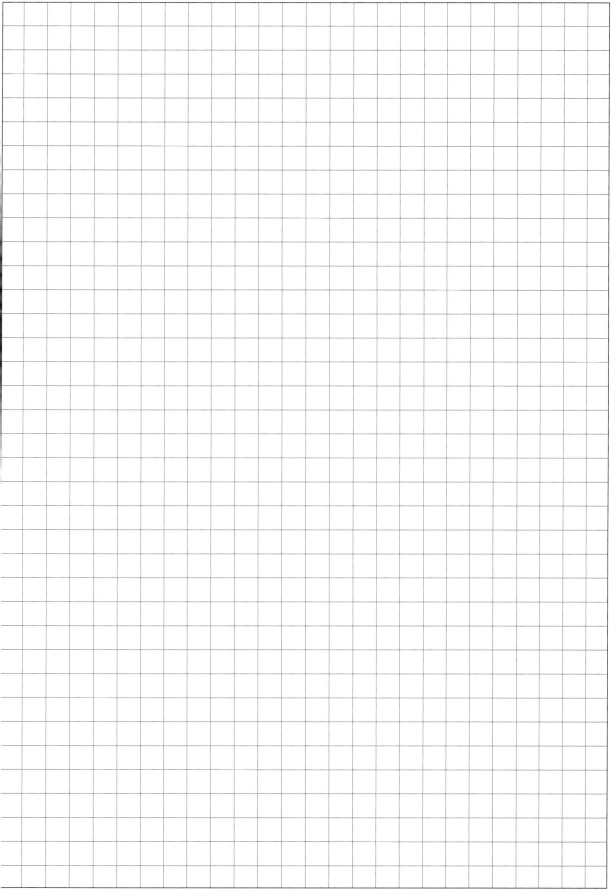

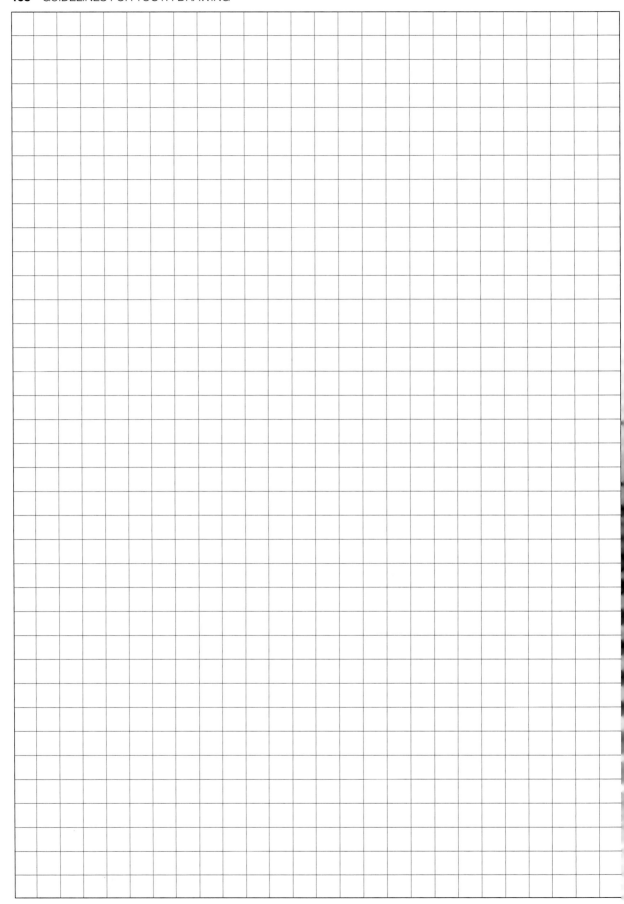

DIMENSIONS OF PERMANENT MANDIBULAR SECOND PREMOLAR*

Cervico-incisal Length of Crown	8.0
Length of Root	14.5
Mesiodistal Diameter of Crown	7.0
Mesiodistal Diameter of CEJ	5.0
Buccolingual Diameter	8.0
Buccolingual Diameter of CEJ	7.0
Curvature of CEJ—Mesial	1.0
Curvature of CEJ—Distal	0.0

*In millimeters; adapted from Nelson SJ: *Wheeler's Dental Anatomy, Physiology, and Occlusions,* ed 9, WB Saunders, Philadelphia, 2009.

CEJ = cementoenamel junction

CHECKLIST FOR PERMANENT MANDIBULAR SECOND PREMOLAR

Features Noted	Features Present
Crown Features	
Usually three cusps present with buccal ridge	
Occlusal table with marginal ridges and cusps, with tips, ridges, inclined planes, and grooves (usually U-shaped groove pattern with increased supplemental grooves), fossae, pits	
Distal marginal ridge more cervically located, so more occlusal surface visible from distal view	
Mesial and distal contact is just cervical to the junction of occlusal and middle thirds	
Root Features	
Single rooted	
Proximal root concavities	

Name _____   Tooth Number/Name _____

Date _____   Instructor Rating _____

DRAWING EVALUATION CHECKLIST

RATING SCALE

Fully Correct = 2 points   Major Error = 0 points
Minor Error = 1 point   Note: NA (non-appropriate)

SELF-EVALUATION RATING

Five Views	Clearly Drawn	Accurate Sizing	General Features Included	Specific Features Included
1. Facial View				
2. Lingual View				
3. Mesial View				
4. Distal View				
5. Incisal/ Occlusal View				

Self-Evaluation Rating $= \dfrac{\text{Points received}}{\text{Points possible}} =$ _____ $=$ _____ %

INSTRUCTOR EVALUATION RATING

Five Views	Clearly Drawn	Accurate Sizing	General Features Included	Specific Features Included
1. Facial View				
2. Lingual View				
3. Mesial View				
4. Distal View				
5. Incisal/ Occlusal View				

Instructor Evaluation Rating $= \dfrac{\text{Points received}}{\text{Points possible}} =$ _____ $=$ _____ %

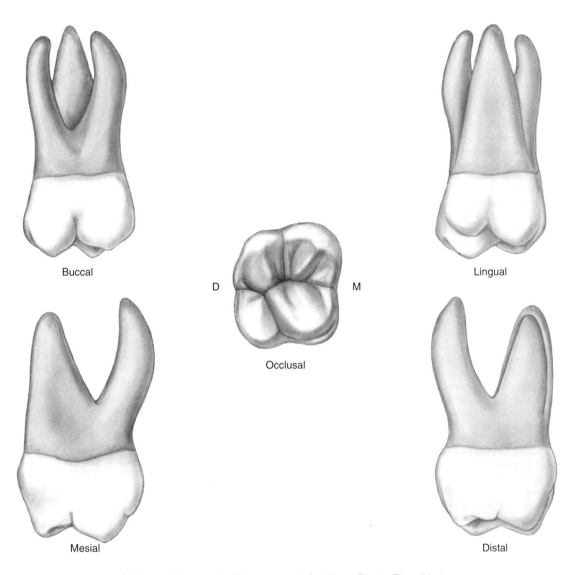

Buccal

Lingual

D   M

Occlusal

Mesial

Distal

Various Views of a Permanent Maxillary Right First Molar

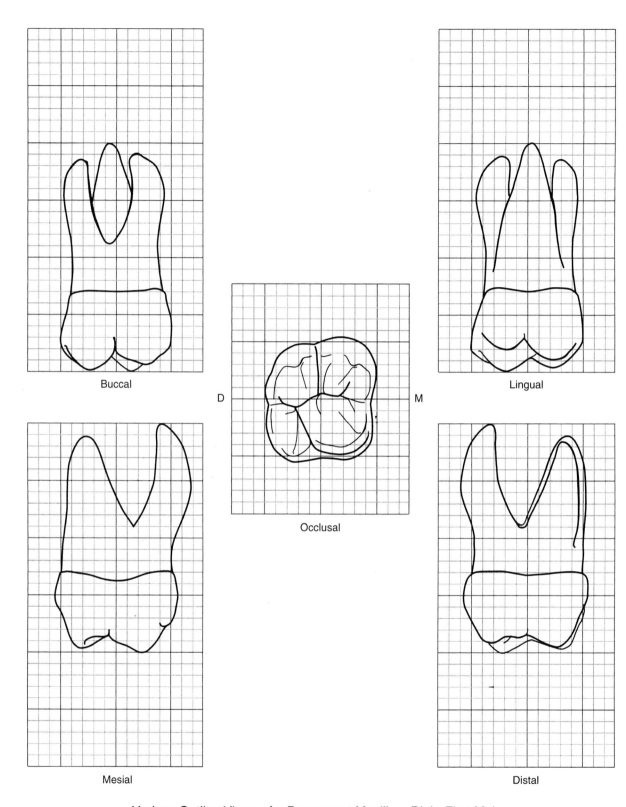

Buccal

D   M

Occlusal

Lingual

Mesial

Distal

Various Outline Views of a Permanent Maxillary Right First Molar

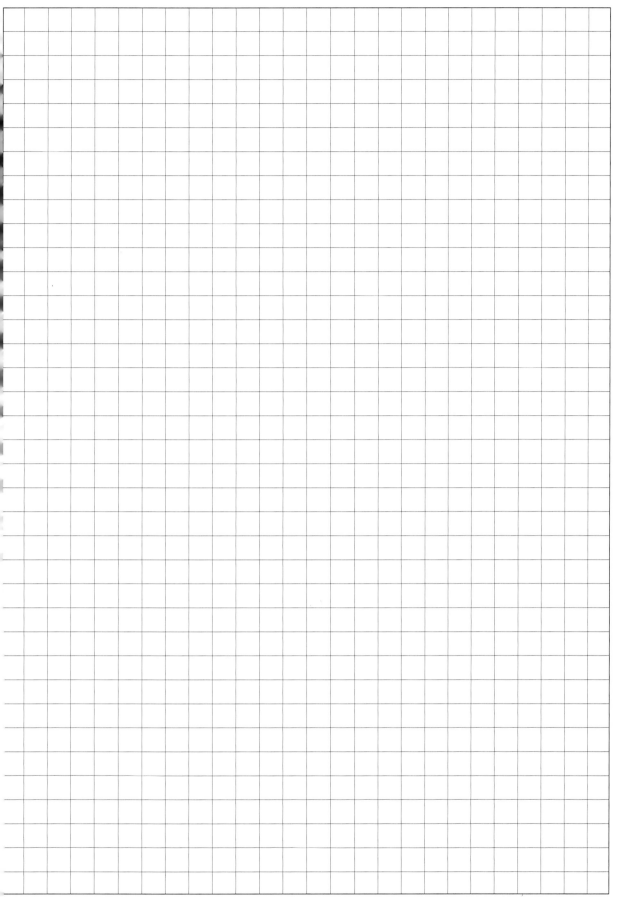

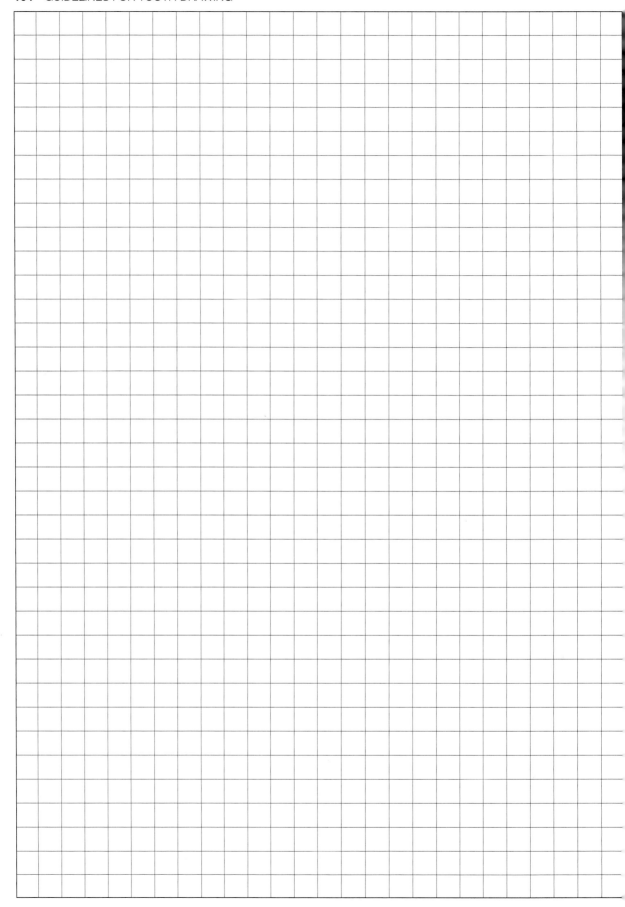

DIMENSIONS OF PERMANENT MAXILLARY FIRST MOLAR*

Cervico-incisal Length of Crown	Buccal: 7.0	Lingual: 6.0
Length of Root	Buccal: 12	Lingual: 13
Mesiodistal Diameter of Crown	10.0	
Mesiodistal Diameter of CEJ	8.0	
Buccolingual Diameter	11.0	
Buccolingual Diameter of CEJ	10.0	
Curvature of CEJ—Mesial	1.0	
Curvature of CEJ—Distal	0.0	

*In millimeters; adapted from Nelson SJ: *Wheeler's Dental Anatomy, Physiology, and Occlusions*, ed 9, WB Saunders, Philadelphia, 2009.

CHECKLIST FOR PERMANENT MAXILLARY FIRST MOLAR

Features Noted	Features Present
Crown Features	
Four major cusps, with buccal cusps almost equal in height and fifth minor cusp of Carabelli associated with mesiolingual cusp and groove	
Buccal cervical ridge	
Mesiolingual cusp outline longer and larger, but not as sharp as distolingual cusp	
Occlusal table with prominent oblique ridge, marginal ridges and cusps, with tips, ridges, inclined planes, and grooves, fossae, pits	
Mesial contact is at junction of occlusal and middle thirds	
Distal contact at middle third	
Root Features	
Trifurcated roots with furcations, root trunks, and root concavities	
Divergent roots with furcations well removed from the CEJ	

Name _____   Tooth Number/Name _____

Date _____   Instructor Rating _____

DRAWING EVALUATION CHECKLIST

RATING SCALE
Fully Correct = 2 points   Major Error = 0 points
Minor Error = 1 point   Note: NA (non-appropriate)

SELF-EVALUATION RATING

Five Views	Clearly Drawn	Accurate Sizing	General Features Included	Specific Features Included
1. Facial View				
2. Lingual View				
3. Mesial View				
4. Distal View				
5. Incisal/ Occlusal View				

Self-Evaluation Rating = $\frac{\text{Points received}}{\text{Points possible}}$ = _____ = _____ %

INSTRUCTOR EVALUATION RATING

Five Views	Clearly Drawn	Accurate Sizing	General Features Included	Specific Features Included
1. Facial View				
2. Lingual View				
3. Mesial View				
4. Distal View				
5. Incisal/ Occlusal View				

Instructor Evaluation Rating = $\frac{\text{Points received}}{\text{Points possible}}$ = _____ = _____ %

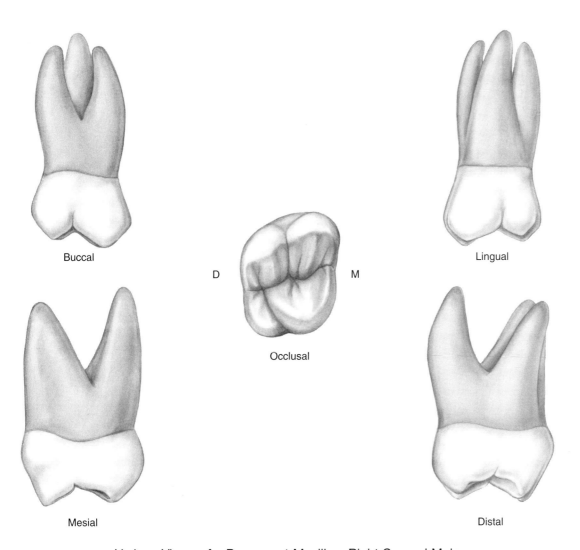

Buccal

Lingual

D   M

Occlusal

Mesial

Distal

Various Views of a Permanent Maxillary Right Second Molar

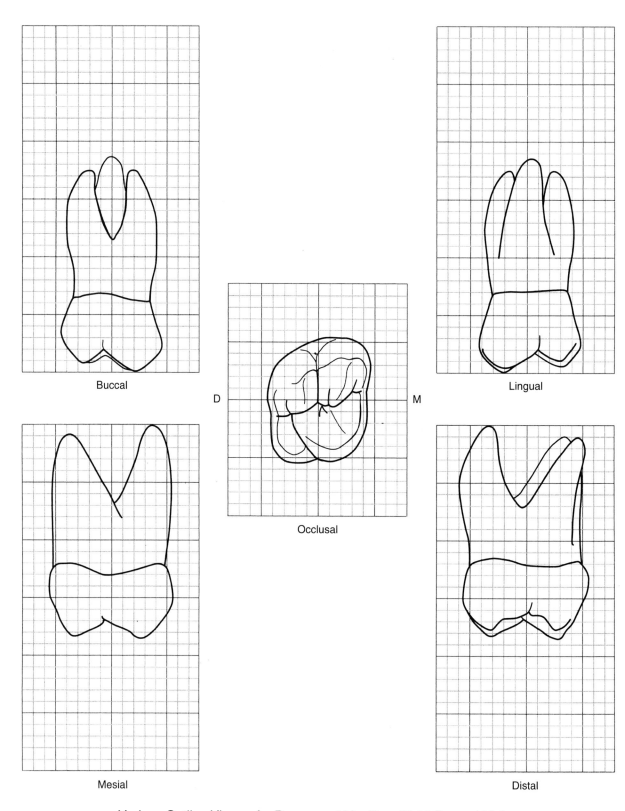

Buccal

D   M

Occlusal

Lingual

Mesial

Distal

Various Outline Views of a Permanent Maxillary Right Second Molar

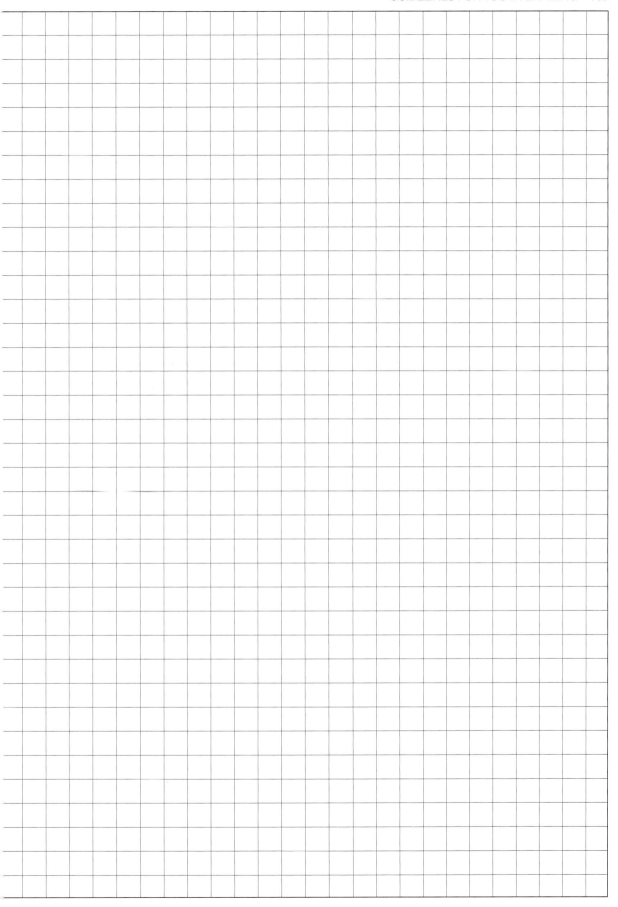

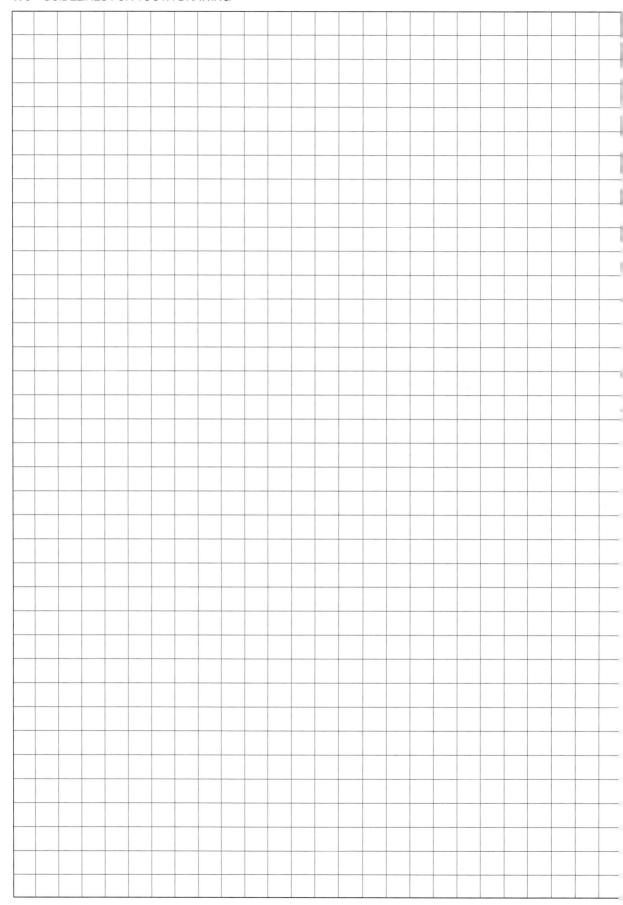

DIMENSIONS OF PERMANENT MAXILLARY SECOND MOLAR*

Cervico-incisal Length of Crown	Buccal:	6.5	Lingual:	5.5
Length of Root	Buccal:	11	Lingual:	12
Mesiodistal Diameter of Crown	9.0			
Mesiodistal Diameter of CEJ	7.0			
Buccolingual Diameter	11.0			
Buccolingual Diameter of CEJ	10.0			
Curvature of CEJ—Mesial	1.0			
Curvature of CEJ—Distal	0.0			

*In millimeters; adapted from Nelson SJ: *Wheeler's Dental Anatomy, Physiology, and Occlusions,* ed 9, WB Saunders, Philadelphia, 2009.

CHECKLIST FOR PERMANENT MAXILLARY FIRST MOLAR

Features Noted	Features Present
Crown Features	
Four cusps usually	
Buccal cervical ridge	
Mesiobuccal cusp longer than distobuccal cusp; distolingual cusp usually smaller	
Occlusal table with less prominent oblique ridge, marginal ridges and cusps, with tips, ridges, inclined planes, and grooves, fossae, pits	
Mesial contact at middle third	
Distal contact at middle third	
Root Features	
Trifurcated roots with furcations, root trunks, and root concavities	
Less divergent roots	

Name _____   Tooth Number/Name _____

Date _____   Instructor Rating _____

DRAWING EVALUATION CHECKLIST

RATING SCALE

Fully Correct = 2 points   Major Error = 0 points
Minor Error = 1 point   Note: NA (non-appropriate)

SELF-EVALUATION RATING

Five Views	Clearly Drawn	Accurate Sizing	General Features Included	Specific Features Included
1. Facial View				
2. Lingual View				
3. Mesial View				
4. Distal View				
5. Incisal/ Occlusal View				

$$\text{Self-Evaluation Rating} = \frac{\text{Points received}}{\text{Points possible}} = \underline{\hspace{3cm}} = \underline{\hspace{2cm}} \%$$

INSTRUCTOR EVALUATION RATING

Five Views	Clearly Drawn	Accurate Sizing	General Features Included	Specific Features Included
1. Facial View				
2. Lingual View				
3. Mesial View				
4. Distal View				
5. Incisal/ Occlusal View				

$$\text{Instructor Evaluation Rating} = \frac{\text{Points received}}{\text{Points possible}} = \underline{\hspace{3cm}} = \underline{\hspace{2cm}} \%$$

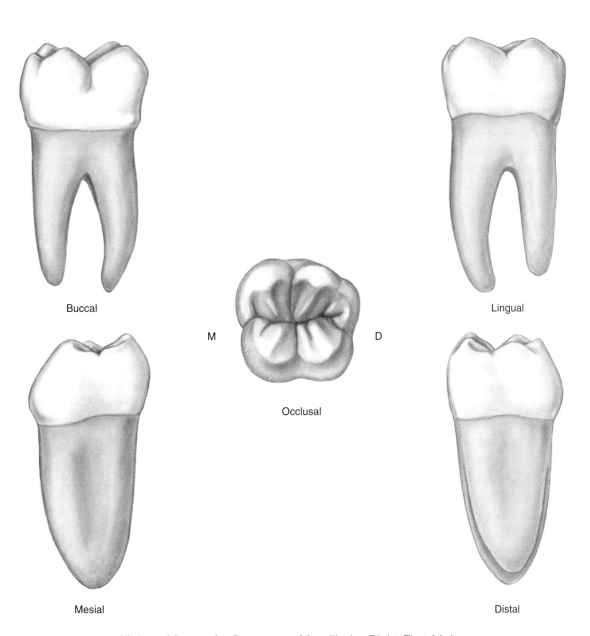

Buccal

Lingual

M

D

Occlusal

Mesial

Distal

Various Views of a Permanent Mandibular Right First Molar

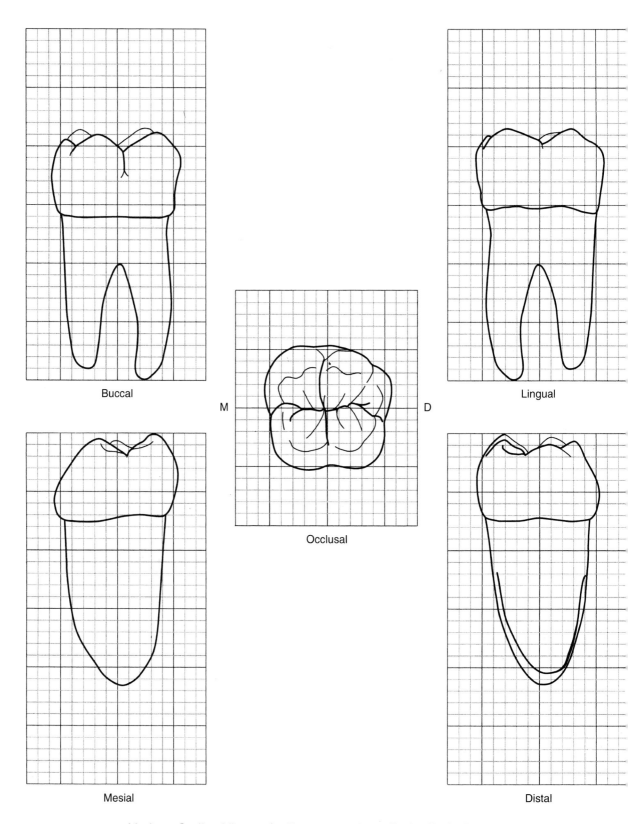

Buccal

M

D

Occlusal

Lingual

Mesial

Distal

Various Outline Views of a Permanent Mandibular Right First Molar

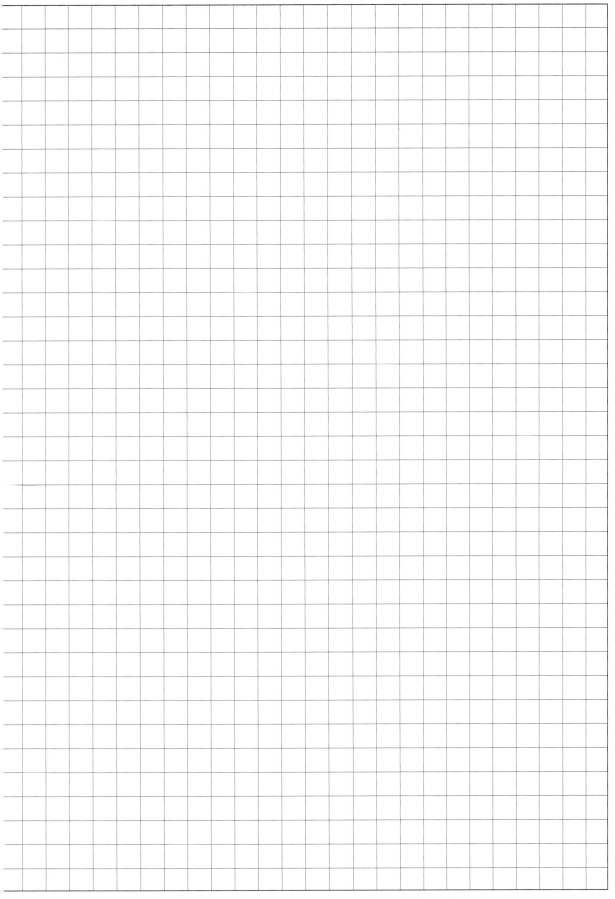

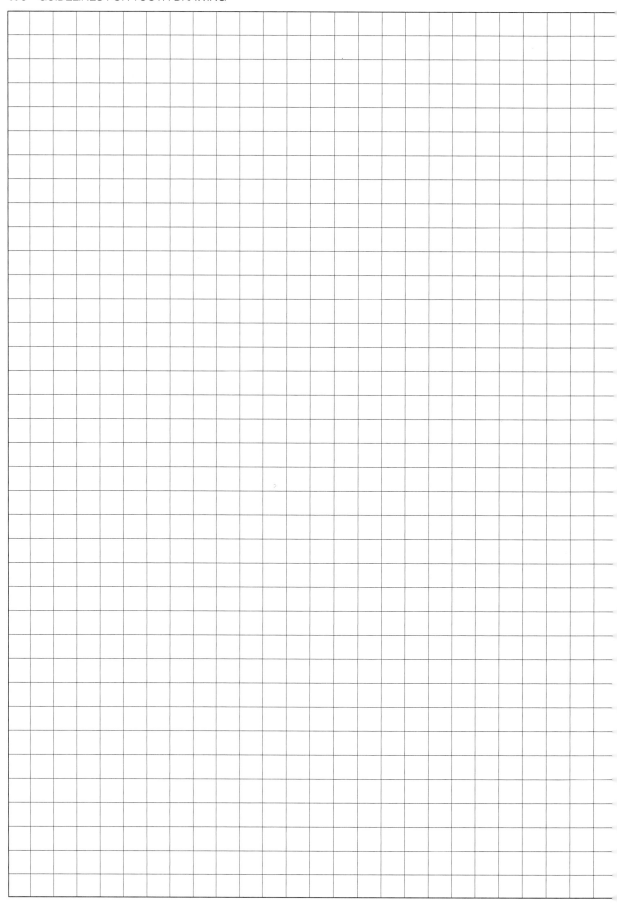

DIMENSIONS OF PERMANENT MANDIBULAR FIRST MOLAR*

Cervico-incisal Length of Crown	7.5
Length of Root	14.0
Mesiodistal Diameter of Crown	11.0
Mesiodistal Diameter of CEJ	9.0
Buccolingual Diameter	10.5
Buccolingual Diameter of CEJ	9.0
Curvature of CEJ—Mesial	1.0
Curvature of CEJ—Distal	0.0

*In millimeters; adapted from Nelson SJ: *Wheeler's Dental Anatomy, Physiology, and Occlusions,* ed 9, WB Saunders, Philadelphia, 2009.

CHECKLIST FOR PERMANENT MANDIBULAR FIRST MOLAR

Features Noted	Features Present
Crown Features	
Five cusps with Y-shaped groove pattern and with buccal groove	
Buccal cervical ridge	
Distal cusp is smallest	
Occlusal table with marginal ridges and cusps, with tips, ridges, inclined planes, and grooves, fossae, pits	
Mesial and distal contact is at junction of occlusal and middle thirds	
Root Features	
Bifurcated roots with furcations, root trunks, and root concavities	
Divergent roots with furcations well removed from the CEJ	

Name _____   Tooth Number/Name _____

Date _____   Instructor Rating _____

DRAWING EVALUATION CHECKLIST

RATING SCALE
Fully Correct = 2 points   Major Error = 0 points
Minor Error = 1 point   Note: NA (non-appropriate)

SELF-EVALUATION RATING

Five Views	Clearly Drawn	Accurate Sizing	General Features Included	Specific Features Included
1. Facial View				
2. Lingual View				
3. Mesial View				
4. Distal View				
5. Incisal/ Occlusal View				

$$\text{Self-Evaluation Rating} = \frac{\text{Points received}}{\text{Points possible}} = \underline{\hspace{2cm}} = \underline{\hspace{1.5cm}} \%$$

INSTRUCTOR EVALUATION RATING

Five Views	Clearly Drawn	Accurate Sizing	General Features Included	Specific Features Included
1. Facial View				
2. Lingual View				
3. Mesial View				
4. Distal View				
5. Incisal/ Occlusal View				

$$\text{Instructor Evaluation Rating} = \frac{\text{Points received}}{\text{Points possible}} = \underline{\hspace{2cm}} = \underline{\hspace{1.5cm}} \%$$

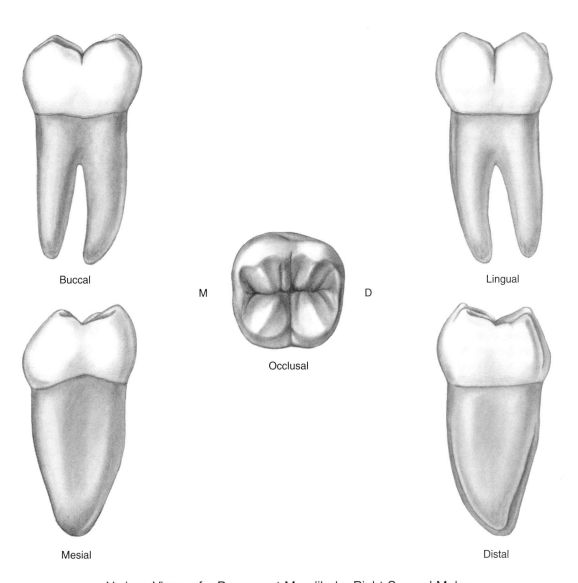

Buccal

M

D

Occlusal

Lingual

Mesial

Distal

Various Views of a Permanent Mandibular Right Second Molar

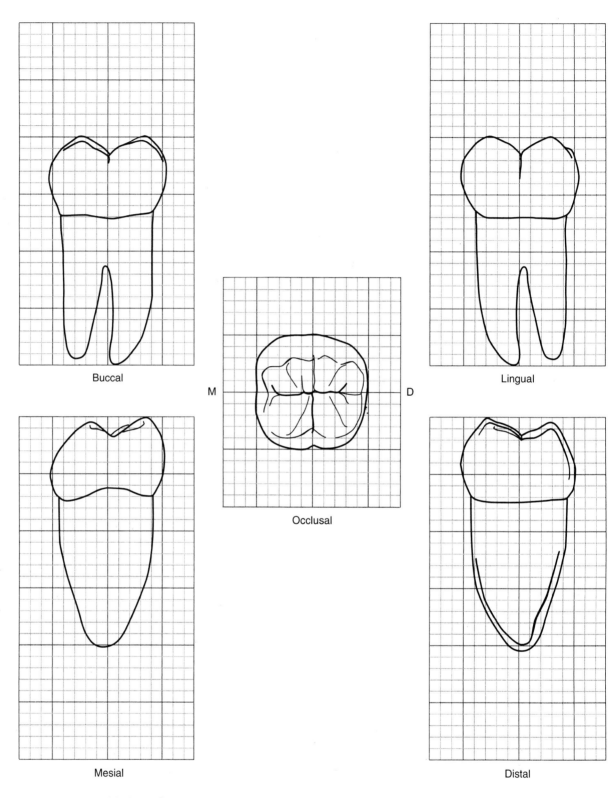

Buccal

Lingual

M   Occlusal   D

Mesial

Distal

Various Outline Views of a Permanent Mandibular Right Second Molar

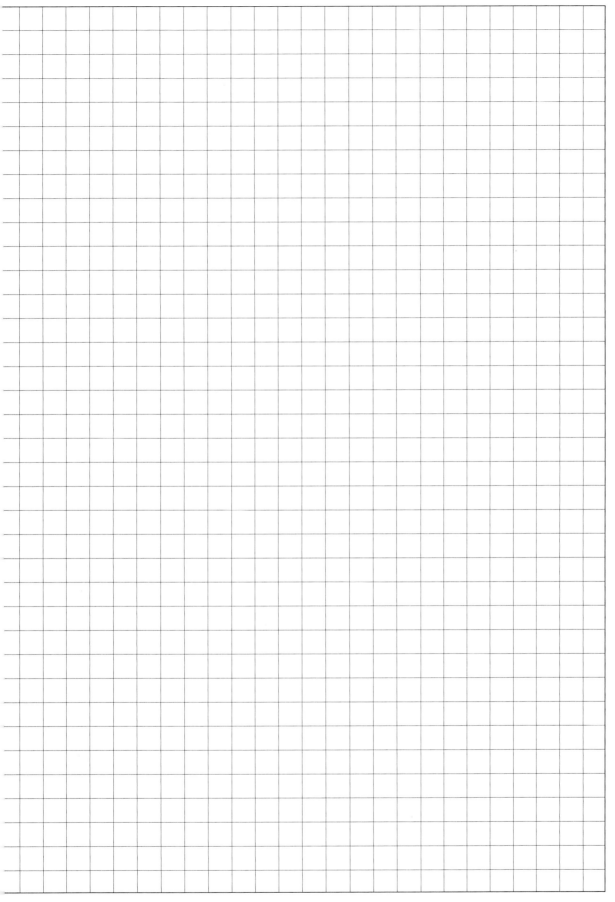

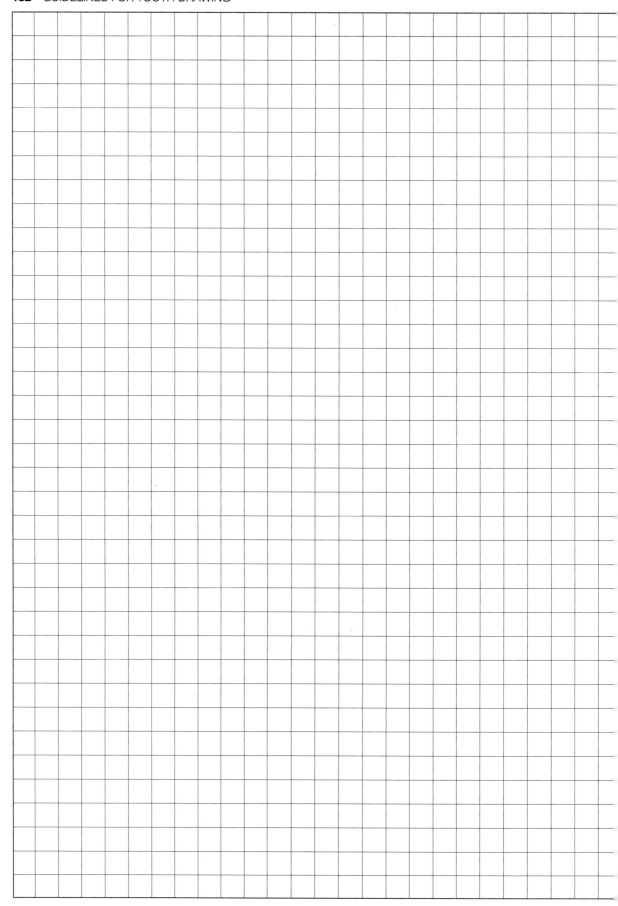

DIMENSIONS OF PERMANENT MANDIBULAR SECOND MOLAR*

Cervico-incisal Length of Crown	7.0
Length of Root	13.0
Mesiodistal Diameter of Crown	10.5
Mesiodistal Diameter of CEJ	8.0
Buccolingual Diameter	10.0
Buccolingual Diameter of CEJ	9.0
Curvature of CEJ—Mesial	1.0
Curvature of CEJ—Distal	0.0

In millimeters; adapted from Nelson SJ: *Wheeler's Dental Anatomy, Physiology, and Occlusions,* ed 9, WB Saunders, Philadelphia, 2009.

CHECKLIST FOR PERMANENT MANDIBULAR SECOND MOLAR

Features Noted	Features Present
Crown Features	
Four cusps with cross-shaped groove pattern	
Buccal cervical ridge	
Wider mesial proximal surface than distal	
Occlusal table with marginal ridges and cusps, with tips, ridges, inclined planes, and grooves, fossae, pits	
Mesial and distal contact is at middle third	
Root Features	
Bifurcated roots with furcations, root trunks, and root concavities	
Less divergent roots with furcations closer to CEJ	

Name _____   Tooth Number/Name _____

Date _____   Instructor Rating _____

DRAWING EVALUATION CHECKLIST

RATING SCALE
Fully Correct = 2 points   Major Error = 0 points
Minor Error = 1 point   Note: NA (non-appropriate)

SELF-EVALUATION RATING

Five Views	Clearly Drawn	Accurate Sizing	General Features Included	Specific Features Included
1. Facial View				
2. Lingual View				
3. Mesial View				
4. Distal View				
5. Incisal/ Occlusal View				

Self-Evaluation Rating = $\frac{\text{Points received}}{\text{Points possible}}$ = _____ = _____ %

INSTRUCTOR EVALUATION RATING

Five Views	Clearly Drawn	Accurate Sizing	General Features Included	Specific Features Included
1. Facial View				
2. Lingual View				
3. Mesial View				
4. Distal View				
5. Incisal/ Occlusal View				

Instructor Evaluation Rating = $\frac{\text{Points received}}{\text{Points possible}}$ = _____ = _____ %

Infection Control for Extracted Teeth: Guidelines and Technique

Guidelines

The use of extracted human teeth in the study of dental anatomy is a valuable addition to the analysis of plastic or plaster teeth. Extracted teeth provide a more realistic form of the anatomy of the tooth; they have more clearly formed cusps, ridges, fossae, and pits. Variations of the ideal tooth form can also be viewed. Extracted teeth can also provide the opportunity to view relatively rare dental anomalies. Although no cases of disease transmitted by extracted teeth have been reported, infection control of the teeth in the teaching laboratory should be a concern. Thus, all dental personnel who collect and inspect extracted teeth should adhere to the infection control procedures. Extracted teeth may be returned to the patients upon request and are not subject to the provisions of the Occupational Safety and Health Administration (OSHA) Bloodborne Pathogens Standard.

OSHA considers extracted teeth to be potentially infectious material. They are sometimes sent to dental laboratories for shade and anatomical comparisons. Occasionally, patients request that their extracted teeth be returned to them. In many instances, extracted teeth will include amalgam restorations. Measures should be taken so that the teeth do not become a source of infection for other people who might come in contact with them. Also, possible pollutants should be taken into consideration because mercury vaporization and exposure is a health hazard. Dispose of extracted teeth as regulated medical waste unless they are returned to the patient or used for study or research (see later guidelines). However, do not dispose of extracted teeth containing amalgam in regulated medical waste intended for incineration.

If kept for study or other purposes, OSHA recommends that "extracted teeth be subject to the containerization and labeling provisions of the bloodborne standard." The Centers for Disease Control and Prevention (CDC) guidelines (1993/2002) state that extracted teeth should be initially collected in a clearly marked with a biohazard symbol and "securely sealed specimen container" (well-constructed, wide-mouthed jar with a secure lid to prevent leakage during transport) with a 10% (diluted 1:10 with tap water) solution of common household bleach (sodium hypochlorite), and then they later can be safely heat-sterilized. The guidelines then specify the use of personal protective equipment when teeth are handled during preparation.

New studies show that teeth also can be soaked in a solution of 10% formalin for two weeks, if desired. However, formalin is a hazardous material identified as a potential carcinogen and should not be used to routinely disinfect amalgam-free teeth. When using formalin, the manufacturer Material Safety Data Sheet (MSDS) should be reviewed for occupational safety and health concerns and to ensure compliance with OSHA recommendations.

It is important to remember that, because of the risk of mercury contamination during tooth preparation, teeth with amalgam cannot be saved or sterilized for viewing. Thus, a documented technique for the infection control of extracted teeth has been updated.*

Technique

Use gloves, mask, and protective eyewear (e.g., wearing appropriate personal protective equipment) during preparation of the teeth. Open collection jars and pour bleach solution into disposal jars, replacing the solution with a new 10% bleach solution. The old solution should be left standing for at least 30 minutes in the disposal jar and then poured into the sewer.

2. Place collected teeth on several layers of paper towels on a tray to protect desktops. Discard collection jars and lids in any trash receptacle.

3. Separate the teeth, and place any teeth to be discarded (such as those with amalgam restorations, if desired) into a wide-mouthed jar with new 10% bleach solution. State and local regulations should be consulted regarding the disposal of amalgam; many metal recycling companies will

---

Technique is modified and permission granted by original author Dr. Thomas M. Schulein, DDS, Associate Professor, University of Iowa, Iowa City, IA (*Journal of Dental Education* 58:6, 1994). The technique has been updated from a research study done by Dominici JT, Eleazer PD, Clark SJ, Staat RH, Scheetz JP: Disinfection/sterilization of extracted teeth for dental students' use (*Journal of Dental Education* 65:11, 2001). The purpose of this study was to determine the effectiveness of different sterilization/disinfection methods for extracted human teeth that were 100% effective in preventing growth by using *Bacillus stearothermophilus*, a bacteria resistant to heat and frequently used to test sterilizers.

accept extracted teeth with amalgam. Contact a recycler and ask about company policies and any specific handling instructions it might have. If extracted teeth containing amalgam restorations are to be used, such as for research purposes, their immersion in 10% formalin solution for 2 weeks has been found to be an effective method of disinfecting both the internal and external structures of the teeth (see earlier note about formalin) without any pollution concerns, but they will still need to handled with precautions (see later note). However, do not use formalin when disinfecting extracted teeth containing amalgam before disposal. Continued research is needed to determine the best method for treating teeth before research activities.

4. Place remaining teeth into clear zipper-lock plastic bag with a new 10% bleach solution. Place closed bag in an ultrasonic for 30 minutes. Solution from the bag is poured down the sewer.

5. Teeth should be covered with a wet paper towel to maintain moisture. Place teeth in plastic autoclave bags, and tape them closed. Heat sterilized teeth in an autoclave for 40 minutes at 240°F and 20 psi. Discard paper towels, plastic bag, and gloves in the biohazard waste receptacle. Spray tray with germicidal detergent, and allow to dry. Thus, autoclaving teeth for preclinical laboratory exercises does not alter their physical properties sufficiently to compromise the learning experience in the laboratory setting. However, autoclave sterilization of extracted teeth does affect dentinal structure enough to compromise dental materials research.

6. Place autoclaved teeth into clear wide-mouthed jars so that teeth can be viewed and then removed with cotton pliers. Jars are then labeled (according to OSHA standards with a biohazard symbol) and then filled with 0.2% thymol solution. Store the teeth under the solution at all times so that they will not dry and crack.

7. As teeth are needed, they can be removed from the jars with cotton pliers and rinsed with tap water, soaked in a container of tap water, and rinsed again. Although extracted teeth can be effectively sterilized, the CDC states that students must still follow standard precautions (e.g., wearing appropriate personal protective equipment) in handling these materials because preclinical educational exercises simulate clinical experiences.

Selected References and Additional Resources

DeWald JP: The use of extracted teeth for in vitro bonding studies: a review of the infection control considerations, *Dent Mater* 13:74-81, 1997.

Dominici JT, Eleazer PD, Clark SJ, Staat RH, Scheetz JP: Disinfection/sterilization of extracted teeth for dental student use, *J Dent Educ* 65:1278-1280, 2001.

Guidelines for Infection Control in Dental Health-Care Settings, 2003, *MMWR Morb Mortal Wkly Rep* 52(RR-17) 1-61, 2003.

Kumar M, Sequeira PS, Peter S, Bhat GK: Sterilization of extracted human teeth for educational use, *Indian J Med Microbiol* 23(4):256-258, 2005.

Lee JJ, Nettey-Marbell A, Cook A, Pimenta LA, Leonard R, Ritter AV: The effect of storage medium and sterilization on dentin bond strengths, *J Am Dent Assoc* 138:1599-1603, 2007.

McGuckin RS, Pashley DH: The effect of disinfection/sterilization treatments on gluma mediated dentin shear bond strengths, *Am J Dent* 3:278-282, 1990.

Pantera EA, Schuster GS: Sterilization of extracted human teeth, *J Dent Educ* 54:283-285, 1990.

Parsell DE, Stewart BM, Barker JR, Nick TG, Karnes L, Johnson RB: The effect of steam sterilization on the physical properties and perceived cutting characteristics of extracted teeth, *J Dent Educ* 62:260-263 1998.

Schulein TM: Infection control for extracted teeth in the teaching laboratory, *J Dent Educ* 58:411-413, 1994.

Shaffer SE, Barkmeier WW, Gwinnett AJ: Effect of disinfection/sterilization on in vitro enamel bonding *J Dent Educ* 49:658-659, 1985.

Tate WH, White RR: Disinfection of human teeth for educational purposes, *J Dent Educ* 55:583-585, 1991.

U.S. Department of Labor, Occupational Safety and Health Administration. 29 CFR Part 1910.1030. Occupational exposure to bloodborne pathogens; needlestick and other sharps injuries; final rule. Federal Register, 66:5317-5325, 2001. Updated from and including 29 CFR Part 1910.1030. Occupational exposure to bloodborne pathogens; final rule. Federal Register, 56:64003-64182, 1991.

U.S. Department of Labor, Occupational Safety and Health Administration. Enforcement procedures for the occupational exposure to bloodborne pathogens. Washington, DC: U.S. Department of Labor, Occupational Safety and Health Administration, 2001. Directive Number. CPL 02–02–069.

White JM, Goodis HE, Marshall SJ, Marshall GW: Sterilization of teeth by gamma radiation, *J Dent Res* 73:1560-1567, 1994.

White RR, Hays GI: Failure of ethylene oxide to sterilize extracted human teeth, *Dent Mater* 11:321-323, 1995.

Xie B, Dickens SH, Giuseppetti AA: Microtensile bond strength of thermally stressed composite-dentin bonds mediated by one-bottle adhesives, *Am J Dent* 15(3):177-184, 2002.

Occlusal
Evaluation

Supplies Needed

The dental professional will need the following supplies for an initial occlusal evaluation of a permanent dentition: dental chair and light, mirror, explorer, probe, hand mirror, articulating paper, floss, an occlusal evaluation form, and personal protection equipment. Explanations of the reasons for taking an occlusal evaluation and how it relates to dental treatment, including the terms used in this evaluation, are located in the associated textbook. In many dental offices, the occlusal evaluation is a part of the periodontal evaluation; newer technology using a transcutaneous electrical nerve stimulation unit for patient relaxation can be included.

Occlusal History and Extraoral and Intraoral Findings

Before performing an occlusal evaluation, take notes on the **occlusal history** of the patient. Note in the chart any removable prostheses (flippers, retainers, night and sports guards, and partial and/or complete dentures), and have the patient keep them in during the evaluation if they are worn regularly. Record any occlusal complaints, habits, and applicable physical or psychological findings from the patient or medical history questionnaire that may be pertinent to the patient's occlusal history. Note these findings under occlusal history.

Additionally, note any information found during an **extraoral examination** that may be pertinent to the patient's occlusion. This includes any facial asymmetries, loss of vertical dimension, mandibular deviation upon opening, and temporomandibular disorder symptoms. Also note any information found during an intraoral examination that may be pertinent to the patient's occlusion. Note any **attrition** of the dentition, and record the location and amount involved in the area provided on the chart. Finally, note any **mobility** of the dentition by circling the involved teeth in red opposite the mobility section.

Record any **sensitivity** to thermal changes or percussion (gentle tapping). Record any deviations in the **intra-arch form or alignment**, such as loss of contact, plunging cusps, open bite, crossbites, and any arch collapse. Note also any missing, rotated, supererupted, or drifted or fractured teeth or those with abfraction, including any changes in restorations because occlusal trauma is the main reason for early restoration failure. Changes in the midline of the two dentitions should also be noted. Note these items related to intra-arch findings in the areas listed on the chart.

Finally, record any pertinent information from a **radiographic examination** of the dentition, such as amount of bone support, alterations of the periodontal ligament, root resorption, non-vital and fixed prosthetic teeth, including veneers, crowns, and implants. Record these findings in the area listed as the radiographic examination.

Achieving Centric Relation and Patient/Clinician Positioning

For the dental professional to evaluate the occlusion of a patient, the patient must be first in centric relation. **Centric relation (CR)** is the end point of closure of the mandible in which the mandible is in the most retruded position. Centric relation is used as a baseline for an occlusal evaluation.

To achieve centric relation, the patient is first placed in an upright position. The patient should be relaxed, looking straight ahead with lips parted. The clinician should be sitting or standing in front and to the side of the patient. The clinician's thumb should be placed against the outside of the chin, with the fingers placed under the inferior border of the mandible to alternately lift and loosen the mandible. The clinician must then establish the hinge movement of the mandible by gently arcing the mandible with the fingers several times in a closing and opening manner. Then, the loosened mandible is guided into closure, where the mandible is placed in its most retruded position.

Determining Angle's Classification of Malocclusion

Once the patient is in centric relation, determine the **Angle's classification of malocclusion** to determine the form of the patient's dentition. Most cases can be placed into three main classes on the basis of the position of the permanent maxillary first molar relative to the mandibular first molar. The position of the canines must also be noted. Additionally, any subgroups within the classification must be noted. The classification is recorded in the area on the chart labeled *Angle's classification*. A tendency to any type of malocclusion can be noted using the molar relationship (less than the width of a premolar).

Measuring Overjet

With the patient maintained in centric relation, **overjet** or horizontal overlap between the two arches is measured in millimeters with the tip of the periodontal probe. The probe is placed at a right angle to the labial surface of a mandibular incisor at the base of the incisal edge of a maxillary incisor. The measurement is taken from the labial surface of the mandibular incisor to the lingual surface of the maxillary incisor. Note that the labiolingual width of the maxillary incisor is not included in the measurement. The overjet is recorded in the chart in the area labeled *overjet*.

Measuring Overbite

Overbite, or vertical overlap between the two arches, is measured in millimeters with the tip of the periodontal probe after the patient is placed in centric relation. The probe is placed on the incisal edge of the maxillary incisor at right angles to the mandibular incisor. As the patient opens the mouth or depresses the jaws, the probe is then placed vertically against the mandibular incisor to measure the distance to the incisal edge of the mandibular incisor. The overbite is recorded in the chart in the area labeled *overbite*.

Checking for Interocclusal Clearance

Allow the patient to rest while checking for **interocclusal clearance**, the space when the mandible is at rest. In this rest position, an average space of 2 to 3mm can be noted between the masticatory surfaces of the maxillary and mandibular teeth. Thus, failure of a patient to assume this position when the jaws are not at work may mean the patient is temporarily tense or has parafunctional habits such as clenching or grinding (bruxism). Interocclusal clearance is measured in millimeters and recorded in the area for it on the chart. If no interocclusal clearance is noted during mandibular rest, follow-up questions may be necessary to ascertain any tension or parafunctional habits.

Checking for Premature Contact

After the patient relaxes for a moment, centric relation is again attained, and the patient is asked where the teeth first touch during occlusion. If it is a lone tooth, the tooth is considered to be part of a **premature contact**. Articulation paper can be used to check for these premature contacts, which limit the opportunity for maximal intercuspation of the teeth. Premature contacts are recorded in the chart by circling the tooth numbers of the contacting teeth in red opposite the centric relation occlusion section.

Achieving Centric Occlusion

Next, have the patient clench the teeth together, and note the amount of slide in millimeters from their position in centric relation to their position in centric occlusion. **Centric occlusion (CO)**, or habitual occlusion, is the voluntary position of the dentition that allows maximal contact when the teeth occlude. Record the amount of slide or shift in millimeters in the chart; the direction of the slide is also recorded (anterior, right, left, posterior). Normally, the amount of slide or shift from CR to CO is about 1mm. If no slide is noted, then position of the teeth in centric relation is the same as in centric occlusion and CR = CO is circled in the chart.

Checking Lateral Occlusion

Next, the patient's occlusion in lateral deviation or excursion must be checked. Evaluation of **lateral occlusion** is made by moving the mandible to either the right or the left until the canines on that side are in **canine rise**, or cuspid rise. The clinician must support the patient's mandible with the operating hand and gently move the mandible into centric relation or even centric occlusion. Then, the clinician slowly guides the mandible to the patient's right or left until the opposing canines are edge to edge.

The side to which the mandible has been moved is the **working side**. There are two working sides noted in an occlusal evaluation: right lateral and left lateral. Before the canines come into contact on each side, other individual teeth that make contact on the working side should be noted. These **working contacts** are recorded by circling the tooth numbers of the contacting teeth in blue on the chart in the area opposite the lateral occlusion section for the appropriate side.

The other side of the arch from the working side during lateral occlusion is the **balancing side**. If any teeth make contact on the opposite or balancing side during lateral occlusion, they are recorded as a **balancing interference** and are circled in red for the appropriate side. If **group function**, where most of the entire posterior quadrant functions during lateral occlusion are present, it should be recorded by circling the tooth numbers of the involved group of teeth in blue on the chart opposite the lateral occlusion section for the appropriate side.

Do not allow patients to move freely into lateral deviation because they may choose a convenient path to bypass an interference. For further confirmation of any balancing interferences during lateral deviation, place floss across the retromolar pads extending out to the labial commissures, or place articulating paper over the occlusal surfaces on the appropriate side. After guiding the patient into either right or left lateral occlusion, the clinician slips the floss or articulating paper forward, noting any points of contact.

Checking Protrusive Occlusion

Finally, the **protrusive occlusion** of the patient must be checked. With the patient's teeth in centric occlusion, the clinician supports the mandible with the operating hand. Have the patient slowly move the mandible forward so that the two dentitions are in an edge-to-edge relationship. Note any posterior/canine contacts or **balancing interferences** during protrusion, and record this information on the chart by circling the contacting teeth in red opposite the protrusive section. Also note the anterior teeth that are in contact during protrusion, or the **working contacts**, by circling on the chart the tooth numbers of the contacting teeth in blue opposite the protrusive section.

For further confirmation of working contacts and any balancing interferences during protrusion, place the floss across the retromolar pads extending out to the labial commissures. Then, guide the patient into protrusive occlusion, and slip the floss forward between the teeth until resistance of contacting teeth is met.

INITIAL OCCLUSAL EXAMINATION

Patient's Name _____ Chart No. _____ Date _____

Occlusal History _____

_____

Extraoral Findings _____

_____

Intraoral Findings _____

_____

Angle's Classification _____ Molar _____ Canine _____ Subgroup

Interocclusal Clearance _____ mm   Sensitivity _____

Overjet _____ mm   Overbite _____ mm   Attrition _____

Intra-arch Form/Alignment _____

_____

Radiographic Examination _____

_____

INITIAL OCCLUSAL FINDINGS		
Centric Relation	1 2 3 4 5 6 7 8	9 10 11 12 13 14 15 16
Occlusion	32 31 30 29 28 27 26 25	24 23 22 21 20 19 18 17
CR = CO	mm shift from CR to CO	anterior right left posterior
Right Lateral	1 2 3 4 5 6 7 8	9 10 11 12 13 14 15 16
Occlusion	32 31 30 29 28 27 26 25	24 23 22 21 20 19 18 17
Left Lateral	1 2 3 4 5 6 7 8	9 10 11 12 13 14 15 16
Occlusion	32 31 30 29 28 27 26 25	24 23 22 21 20 19 18 17
Protrusive	1 2 3 4 5 6 7 8	9 10 11 12 13 14 15 16
Occlusion	32 31 30 29 28 27 26 25	24 23 22 21 20 19 18 17
Mobility	1 2 3 4 5 6 7 8	9 10 11 12 13 14 15 16
	32 31 30 29 28 27 26 25	24 23 22 21 20 19 18 17

Unit

Case

Studies

UNIT II: CASE STUDY 1

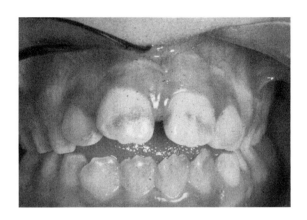

Age	23 years	Scenario
Sex	☐ Male ☒ Female	She visits the dentist regularly every 6 months. Now she is having difficulty with oral hygiene on her small teeth. She regularly chews sugared gum and she does not live now in a water-fluoridated region. Clinical photograph of her dentition was taken. She says she has always had staining on her teeth. Her previous dentist recommended full coverage crowns but said that she needed to wait until the teeth were fully erupted. She also used to suck her thumb when she was a child. When younger, she briefly lived in an area with naturally high levels of fluoride in the drinking water.
Height	5 feet, 8 inches	
Weight	120 pounds	
BP	85/65	
Chief Complaint	"Can we whiten my front teeth?"	
Medical History	None	
Current Medications	Birth control pills	
Social History	First-grade teacher	

1. What is the dental disturbance that is present in the anterior teeth?
   A. Concrescence
   B. Enamel dysplasia
   C. Dentinal dysplasia
   D. Chronic pulpitis

2. To cause this staining, which cell population was mainly disturbed by the high levels of fluoride?
   A. Odontoblasts
   B. Fibroblasts
   C. Ameloblasts
   D. Cementoblasts

3. During what stage(s) of tooth development does this disturbance occur?
   A. Bud stage
   B. Initiation stage
   C. Cap or bell stage
   D. Apposition and maturation stages

4. What type of staining is present in this patient?
   A. Extrinsic
   B. Intrinsic
   C. Transient
   D. Temporary

5. Because the patient has an open bite, what is also present on the incisal edges of the mandibular anterior teeth?
   A. Attrition
   B. Perikymata
   C. Mamelons
   D. Occlusal table

CASE STUDY 2

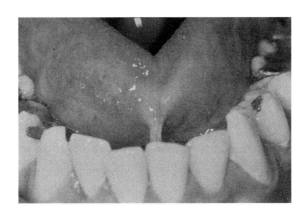

Age	52 years	Scenario
Sex	☒ Male ☐ Female	He has a moderate speech impediment since childhood but never had speech lessons or any surgical procedures, even though they were both suggested to his parents. Mandibular anteriors show crowding and moderate amounts of supragingival calculus.
Height	5 feet 10 inches	
Weight	224 pounds	
BP	115/82	
Chief Complaint	"My lower teeth are getting more crowded."	
Medical History	Repaired right knee	
Current Medications	None	
Social History	Historian at local university	

1. What developmental disturbance is present with this patient?
   A. Gemination
   B. Fusion
   C. Ankyloglossia
   D. Cleft uvula

2. This developmental disturbance involves what portion of the oral cavity?
   A. Lingual frenum
   B. Lingual gingiva
   C. Soft palate
   D. Soft tissues of tongue

3. What week of prenatal development does the tongue begin its specific development?
   A. First week
   B. Second week
   C. Third week
   D. Fourth week

4. The median lingual sulcus noted on the patient's tongue is a superficial demarcation of the fusion of what pair of swellings?
   A. Lateral lingual
   B. Copula
   C. Epiglottic
   D. Tuberculum impar

5. During what prenatal developmental time does the tongue finish the fusion of its swellings?
   A. Fetal period
   B. Embryonic period
   C. Initiation stage
   D. Maturation stage

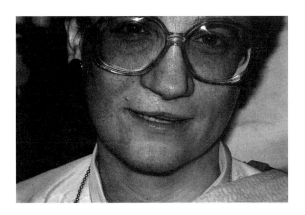

Age	45 years	Scenario
Sex	☐ Male ☒ Female	She had surgery on her left lip from a birth defect as a young child. Had speech lessons as child but is still embarrassed by her slight speech impediment as well as the slight scarring on her upper left lip. No defects noted in her oral cavity. Has moderate inflammation of the maxillary arch and does admit to mouth breathing. Moderate amounts of supragingival calculus noted throughout. Signs of slight to moderate xerostomia and hyposalivation.
Height	5 feet 3 inches	
Weight	105 pounds	
BP	105/68	
Chief Complaint	"Why do I have so much tartar on my teeth?"	
Medical History	Premenopausal and allergy to pollens; past smoker	
Current Medications	Decongestants and short-term hormone replacement therapy	
Social History	Mother of six children	

1. Which of the following developmental disturbances has affected this patient?
   A. Fusion
   B. Cleft palate
   C. Cleft lip
   D. Spina bifida

2. Which of the following processes is involved in this developmental disturbance?
   A. Maxillary process
   B. Lateral nasal process
   C. Mandibular process
   D. Frontonasal process

3. This occurs more commonly and more severely in which of the following populations?
   A. Men
   B. Women
   C. Adolescent group
   D. Geriatric group

4. Which of the following statements is correct concerning this developmental disturbance?
   A. Hereditary in etiology only
   B. May be associated with other abnormalities
   C. Can be found unilaterally only
   D. Occurs mainly on the right side

5. During which prenatal developmental time does this disturbance occur?
   A. Pre-implantation period
   B. Embryonic period
   C. Initiation stage
   D. Apposition stage

CASE STUDY 4

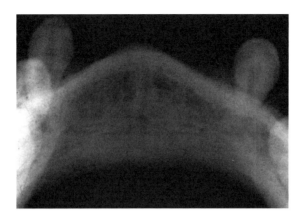

Age	23 years	Scenario
Sex	☒ Male ☐ Female	He appears older than he is because his hair is sparse. He is unable to tolerate a warm environment and needs special measures to keep a normal body temperature since birth. He is saving to have implants placed through a reduced fee program at the local dental school.
Height	6 feet 3 inches	
Weight	165 pounds	
BP	112/84	
Chief Complaint	"I need an assessment for implant placement."	
Medical History	Hearing difficulty due to genetic defect	
Current Medications	None	
Social History	Aspiring actor after finishing high school drama with honors	

1. Which of the following developmental disturbances is present with this patient?
   A. Fetal alcohol syndrome
   B. Down syndrome
   C. Ectodermal dysplasia
   D. Spina bifida

2. Which of the following can be noted in these cases?
   A. Various levels of intellectual disability
   B. Indistinct philtrum and thin upper lip
   C. Abnormalities of skin, hair, nails
   D. Epicanthic folds around eyes

3. This developmental disturbance has which of the following etiological bases?
   A. Teratogenic
   B. Hereditary
   C. Radiation
   D. Drug usage

4. What can be used to help this patient for both cosmetic and functional purposes?
   A. Wheelchair
   B. Dentures
   C. Surgical removal
   D. Speech therapy

5. The embryonic layer involved with this disturbance is formed during which prenatal developmental time?
   A. Fetal period
   B. Embryonic period
   C. Initiation stage
   D. Maturation stage

CASE STUDY 5

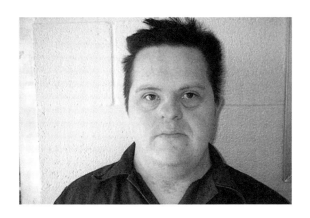

Age	26 years	Scenario
Sex	☒ Male ☐ Female	He has regular appointments set up with the dental office as he does with his speech therapist. He has microdontia and malformed teeth in an oral cavity with undersized bone structure. The roots of his teeth are small and conical, and he mouth breathes. He has moderate early bone loss with chronic periodontal disease and xerostomia.
Height	5 feet 4 inches	
Weight	225 pounds	
BP	110/85	
Chief Complaint	"Need teeth cleaned"	
Medical History	Sleep apnea and hypothyroidism related to genetic disturbance	
Current Medications	Thyroid hormone and anti-seizure medication	
Social History	Lives at group home after being home schooled and works part time at library	

1. Which of the following developmental disturbances is present with this patient?
   A. Fetal alcohol syndrome
   B. Down syndrome
   C. Ectodermal dysplasia
   D. Spina bifida

2. During what prenatal developmental event does this disturbance occur?
   A. Meiosis
   B. Mitosis
   C. Maturation stage
   D. Mesoderm formation

3. What was involved during this developmental disturbance?
   A. Ectopic pregnancy
   B. Infective teratogen
   C. Trisomy 21
   D. Neural tube defect

4. Which of the following may be present with this patient?
   A. Fissures of the tongue
   B. Enlarged tongue
   C. Hyperplasia of the lingual papillae
   D. Furrowed upper lip

5. Which of the following is the correct number of chromosomes present after the joining of the sperm and ovum?
   A. 12
   B. 23
   C. 46
   D. 92

UNIT III: CASE STUDY 1

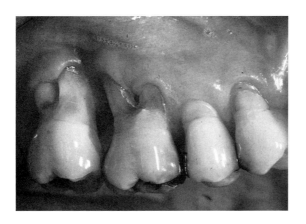

Age	57 years	Scenario
Sex	☐ Male ☒ Female	She regularly visited the dentist until her dentist retired 15 years ago. Diagnosed with chronic periodontal disease (periodontitis), a clinical photograph was taken of both sides of the mouth, along with a complete set of radiographs. Exposed roots were noted throughout, with moderate to severe bone loss. Slight bleeding and moderate mobility were observed throughout. She notes that her teeth are slightly loose.
Height	5 feet 11 inches	
Weight	190 pounds	
BP	102/78	
Chief Complaint	"Why are my teeth so long?"	
Medical History	Past history of skin cancer	
Current Medications	None	
Social History	Retired tennis player	

1. What type of bone has the patient lost between the roots of her molars?
   A. Basal bone
   B. Alveolar crest bone
   C. Interdental septum
   D. Interradicular septum

2. What fiber group of the periodontal ligament is the initial group to be affected by periodontal disease in this patient?
   A. Alveolar crest group
   B. Horizontal group
   C. Oblique group
   D. Apical group

3. The patient's lost alveolar bone and altered periodontal ligament are considered part of which of the following anatomical structures?
   A. Periodontium
   B. Alveolodental ligament
   C. Principal fiber groups
   D. Temporomandibular apparatus

4. What portion of each of the posterior teeth was initially lost as a result of the root exposure?
   A. Predentin
   B. Secondary dentin
   C. Cellular cementum
   D. Coronal enamel

5. Which cell population has been active in removing the alveolar bone in the patient?
   A. Ameloblast
   B. Osteoclast
   C. Odontoblast
   D. Odontoclast

CASE STUDY 2

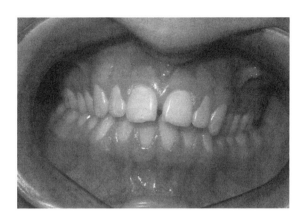

Age	32 years	Scenario
Sex	☒ Male ☐ Female	He has not been to the dentist in 5 years. His previous dentist told him that he needed to brush more. A clinical photograph was taken of both sides of the mouth, along with a complete set of radiographs. Moderate bleeding is noted, but no bone loss was noted on radiographs. He does not regularly brush or floss his teeth and does not routinely take his medication or test his blood.
Height	5 feet 11 inches	
Weight	280 pounds	
BP	110/85	
Chief Complaint	"Why do my teeth bleed when I floss?"	
Medical History	Type II diabetes mellitus	
Current Medications	Oral diabetes medication	
Social History	Real estate agent with four children	

1. What type of mucosa is involved in the inflammation noted in the patient?
   A. Lining mucosa
   B. Specialized mucosa
   C. Masticatory mucosa
   D. Paranasal mucosa

2. Which fiber group of the periodontal ligament is the initial group to be affected with inflammation in this patient?
   A. Gingival fiber group
   B. Alveolar crest group
   C. Horizontal group
   D. Oblique group

3. What is the main underlying cause of this patient's gingival bleeding when flossing?
   A. Thickening of the junctional epithelium
   B. Repair of the lamina propria's blood vessels
   C. Increased blood vessels in the lamina propria
   D. Increased collagen production around blood vessels

4. What is the name given to the patient's present periodontal condition?
   A. Active gingivitis
   B. Chronic gingivitis
   C. Active periodontitis
   D. Chronic periodontitis

5. What is the histological picture of this patient in both the epithelium and lamina propria at the dentogingival junction?
   A. Smooth interface
   B. Decreased numbers of white blood cells
   C. Formation of rete pegs and papillae
   D. All signs of chronic inflammation

CASE STUDY 3

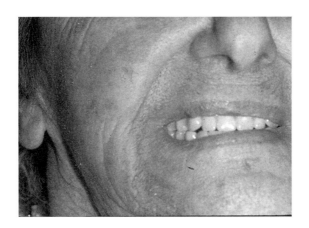

Age	82 years	Scenario
Sex	☐ Male ☒ Female	She is seeing the dentist for the first time after entering the extended care facility. Moderate xerostomia is noted in her mouth. Her maxillary and mandibular complete dentures do not fit comfortably.
Height	5 feet 3 inches	
Weight	112 pounds	
BP	95/78	
Chief Complaint	"Why is my mouth so dry?"	
Medical History	Early stages of Alzheimer's disease; used to smoke	
Current Medications	Antidepressants	
Social History	Former nurse for Red Cross	

1. What is the term used for dry mouth?
   A. Erosion
   B. Abfraction
   C. Hyposalivation
   D. Xerostomia

2. Which is the largest salivary gland in the patient?
   A. Parotid
   B. Submandibular
   C. Sublingual
   D. Von Ebner's

3. What salivary gland usually produces the most saliva?
   A. Parotid
   B. Submandibular
   C. Sublingual
   D. Von Ebner's

4. What portion of the jaws is still completely present in this patient?
   A. Basal bone
   B. Alveolar bone
   C. Interdental septum
   D. Interradicular septum

5. The patient is experiencing diminished length of the lower third of the face; what is this called?
   A. Increase in facial Golden Proportions
   B. Loss of vertical dimension
   C. Partially edentulous state
   D. Mesial drift and supereruption

CASE STUDY 4

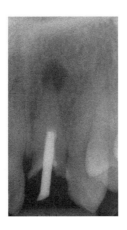

Age	45 years	Scenario
Sex	☒ Male ☐ Female	When he was in his twenties, the affected tooth was treated with root canal surgery because of a dental anomaly. He is experiencing pain on percussion when chewing in the area. A radiograph of the involved tooth was taken. An abscess at the apex of the tooth was noted. He has noted a bad taste in the mouth but no longer chews spit tobacco.
Height	6 feet 4 inches	
Weight	180 pounds	
BP	100/62	
Chief Complaint	"Can you fix my painful broken tooth?"	
Medical History	Osteoarthritis in knees	
Current Medications	Over-the-counter herbal preparations	
Social History	High school basketball coach	

1. What is the dental anomaly that was present in this tooth?
   A. Fusion
   B. Gemination
   C. Dens in dente
   D. Peg lateral

2. Why is the patient experiencing pain with this tooth?
   A. Secondary dentin is filling pulp chamber
   B. Inflammatory edema is pressing on nerves
   C. Inert material is extruding from the pulp
   D. Apical bone is forming at the apex

3. Why did the tooth break in the patient?
   A. Darkening of the tooth
   B. Failure at lobular division
   C. Loss of tooth vitality
   D. Placement of gutta-percha

4. What is the main path by which infection from the pulp travels to the surrounding apical periodontium and causes an abscess?
   A. Apical foramen
   B. Pulp horns
   C. Accessory canals
   D. Dentinal tubules

5. Which cell population can be called upon to produce additional pulp tissue after an injury such as the one this patient has experienced?
   A. Odontoblasts
   B. Red blood cells
   C. White blood cells
   D. Undifferentiated mesenchymal cells

CASE STUDY 5

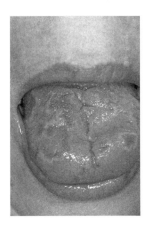

Age	32 years	Scenario
Sex	☐ Male ☒ Female	She is a recent emigrant and regularly visited her dentist. She now uses an electric toothbrush. A clinical photograph of her tongue was taken. She says she has always had this condition of the dorsal surface of the tongue with soreness noted. She brushes her tongue regularly as directed but does not know why this keeps occurring.
Height	5 feet 2 inches	
Weight	120 pounds	
BP	90/78	
Chief Complaint	"Why does the top of my tongue look funny?"	
Medical History	Osteoporosis	
Current Medications	Calcium supplements	
Social History	Chef in restaurant	

1. What is the condition noted on the patient's dorsal surface of the tongue?
   A. Fissured tongue
   B. Central papillary atrophy
   C. Geographic tongue
   D. Burning mouth syndrome

2. What lingual papillae are involved in this tongue condition?
   A. Filiform
   B. Fungiform
   C. Circumvallate
   D. Foliate

3. What type of oral mucosa is on the dorsal surface of the tongue?
   A. Masticatory
   B. Lining
   C. Specialized
   D. Paranasal

4. Which of the following is associated with sensory neuron processes when the patient is working?
   A. Taste pore
   B. Taste cells
   C. Supporting cells
   D. Surrounding tongue epithelium

5. What area of the patient's tongue does not have any fungiform lingual papillae?
   A. Sulcus terminalis
   B. Apex or tip of tongue
   C. Dorsal surface
   D. Near filiform lingual papillae

UNIT IV: CASE STUDY 1

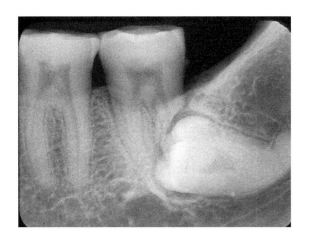

Age	25 years	Scenario
Sex	☒ Male ☐ Female	He had orthodontic treatment as an adolescent. He wears a night guard at night because of bruxism and early symptoms of temporomandibular joint disorder. A periapical radiograph was taken of the sore area of the jaw. No lesions in the mouth were noted. He has generalized moderate attrition. He has a low risk of caries.
Height	6 feet 1 inch	
Weight	190 pounds	
BP	98/67	
Chief Complaint	"Why does my jaw hurt more even with my guard?"	
Medical History	None	
Current Medications	None	
Social History	Professor of chemistry	

1. What is the painful condition noted on the patient's radiograph?
   A. Cyst formation
   B. Microdontia
   C. Partial anodontia
   D. Impacted third molar

2. Which of the following are features of the tooth that is causing the patient's discomfort?
   A. Three roots
   B. Four pulp horns
   C. Consistent crown form
   D. Square crown outline

3. When does the tooth that is causing the patient's discomfort usually complete its roots?
   A. 10-14 years
   B. 13-17 years
   C. 17-21 years
   D. 18-25 years

4. What are the opaque structures noted in the pulp chambers of some of the mandibular posterior teeth?
   A. Denticles
   B. Pulp stones
   C. Sialoliths
   D. Enamel pearls

5. Which structure is located on the patient's temporal bone anterior to the articular fossa of the temporomandibular joint?
   A. Joint capsule
   B. Articular eminence
   C. Synovial membrane
   D. Articulating surface of the condyle

CASE STUDY 2

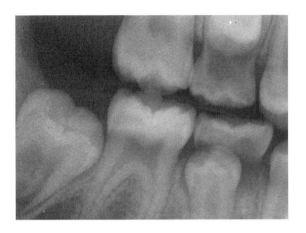

Age	11 years	Scenario
Sex	☒ Male ☐ Female	He has been to the dentist once before at age 7, and dental sealants were placed on all erupted permanent posterior teeth. A bitewing radiograph was taken on both sides of the mouth. Four posterior teeth are loose, and four teeth are partially erupted. Inflammation is noted around loose and partially erupted teeth.
Chief Complaint	"Why do my back teeth feel real loose?"	
Medical History	None	
Current Medications	None	
Social History	Likes to play baseball, wants to be a firefighter	

1. On which teeth were enamel sealants probably placed at the last dental appointment?
   A. First premolars
   B. Second premolars
   C. First molars
   D. Second molars

2. Which partially erupted teeth may need to have enamel sealants placed at the next appointment because of their risk of caries?
   A. First premolars
   B. Second premolars
   C. First molars
   D. Second molars

3. Which of the following teeth may be loose and ready to be exfoliated?
   A. S
   B. T
   C. #2
   D. #30

4. The crown of which permanent posterior tooth appears similar to the crown anatomy of one of the loose teeth?
   A. S
   B. T
   C. #2
   D. #30

5. Which of the following teeth may have already been exfoliated?
   A. S
   B. T
   C. #2
   D. #30

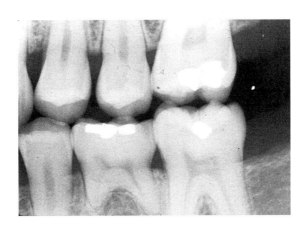

Age	25 years	Scenario
Sex	☐ Male ☒ Female	She is a new patient. At age 6, dental sealants were placed on four teeth that were later restored. She had four permanent posterior teeth extracted at age 13 because of extensive caries and four more at age 20 because of impaction. Her most recent dentist told her that some of her "adult" teeth were never going to erupt. A bitewing radiograph was taken on both sides of the mouth. A small posterior tooth was noted on both sides of the mouth. She is having difficulty with oral hygiene care on her smaller teeth. She regularly chews sugared gum and does not live in a water-fluoridated region.
Height	5 feet 6 inches	
Weight	180 pounds	
BP	98/75	
Chief Complaint	"Why is one of my back teeth on each side smaller than the rest?"	
Medical History	None	
Current Medications	None	
Social History	Hairdresser with three small children	

1. For which posterior tooth does the patient exhibit partial anodontia?
   A. Second premolars
   B. First molars
   C. Second molars
   D. Third molars

2. Which posterior teeth did the patient have extracted as an adolescent?
   A. Second premolars
   B. First molars
   C. Second molars
   D. Third molars

3. Which posterior teeth did the patient have extracted as a young adult?
   A. Second premolars
   B. First molars
   C. Second molars
   D. Third molars

4. Which posterior permanent teeth have been restored in the patient?
   A. Second premolars
   B. First molars
   C. Second molars
   D. Third molars

5. Of the teeth present in the patient, which of following teeth have two roots?
   A. Second premolars
   B. First molars
   C. Second molars
   D. Third molars

CASE STUDY 4

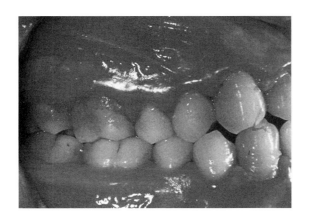

Age	42 years	Scenario
Sex	☒ Male ☐ Female	He had orthodontics as a teenager but did not wear a retainer as suggested. Third molars were extracted at age 20. He undergoes bruxism at night. He has not visited a dentist in 12 years. No caries were noted. A clinical photograph was taken of both sides of the mouth, along with a complete set of radiographs. Moderate inflammation of the gingiva is present, with deposits noted throughout. He has always used a soft toothbrush and gargled with medicated mouth rinses.
Height	5 feet 10 inches	
Weight	180 pounds	
BP	115/95	
Chief Complaint	"Why are my bottom eye teeth sensitive at the gumline when I drink coffee?"	
Medical History	Smokes and has high blood pressure controlled with medication.	
Current Medications	Diuretics	
Social History	Writer of science fiction	

1. What is Angle's classification of the patient's posterior dentition on the right side?
   A. Class I
   B. Class II, division I
   C. Class II, division II
   D. Class III

2. What other occlusal evaluation notes can be made regarding the right side of the dentition?
   A. Severe crossbite
   B. Open bite
   C. Severe overjet
   D. End-to-end bite

3. What may be occurring on the patient's lower teeth to make them sensitive to hot fluids?
   A. Erosion
   B. Abfraction
   C. Pulpitis
   D. Toothbrush abrasion

4. What is the correct term used for grinding the teeth?
   A. Clenching
   B. Xerostomia
   C. Bruxism
   D. Passive eruption

5. What part of the anatomy of the tooth is initially lost with bruxism?
   A. Fossae
   B. Pits
   C. Fissures
   D. Cusps